SECOND EDITION

Practical Guide to Exercise Physiology

D0879106

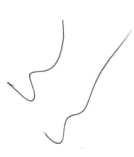

SECOND EDITION

Practical Guide to Exercise Physiology

THE SCIENCE OF EXERCISE TRAINING AND PERFORMANCE NUTRITION

Bob Murray, PhD

Sports Science Insights, LLC

W. Larry Kenney, PhD

Pennsylvania State University

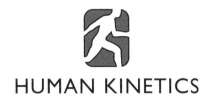

HUMAN KINETICS

Library of Congress Cataloging-in-Publication Data

Names: Murray, Robert, 1949- author. | Kenney, W. Larry, author.
Title: Practical guide to exercise physiology : the science of exercise
 training and performance nutrition / Bob Murray, PhD, Sports Science
 Insights, LLC W. Larry Kenney, PhD, Pennsylvania State University,
 University Park.
Description: Second edition. | Champaign, IL : Human Kinetics, Inc., [2021]
 | Includes index.
Identifiers: LCCN 2020016043 (print) | LCCN 2020016044 (ebook) | ISBN
 9781492599050 (paperback) | ISBN 9781492599067 (epub) | ISBN
 9781492599081 (pdf)
Subjects: LCSH: Exercise--Physiological aspects. | Exercise--Technique.
Classification: LCC RA781 .M775 2021 (print) | LCC RA781 (ebook) | DDC
 613.7/1--dc23
LC record available at https://lccn.loc.gov/2020016043
LC ebook record available at https://lccn.loc.gov/2020016044

ISBN: 978-1-4925-9905-0

Senior Acquisitions Editor: Amy N. Tocco; **Senior Developmental Editor:** Christine M. Drews; **Managing Editor:** Julia R. Smith; **Copyeditor:** Pamela S. Johnson; **Indexer:** Nan N. Badgett; **Permissions Manager:** Dalene Reeder; **Graphic Designer:** Sean Roosevelt; **Cover Designer:** Keri Evans; **Cover Design Specialist:** Susan Rothermel Allen; **Photograph (cover):** Matt Lincoln/Cultura/Getty Images; **Photographs (interior):** © Human Kinetics, unless otherwise noted; **Photo Asset Manager:** Laura Fitch; **Photo Production Manager:** Jason Allen; **Senior Art Manager:** Kelly Hendren; **Illustrations:** © Human Kinetics, unless otherwise noted; **Printer:** Walsworth

Printed in the United States of America   10 9 8 7 6 5 4 3 2 1

The paper in this book was manufactured using responsible forestry methods.

Human Kinetics
1607 N. Market Street
Champaign, IL 61820
USA

United States and International
Website: **US.HumanKinetics.com**
Email: info@hkusa.com
Phone: 1-800-747-4457

Canada
Website: **Canada.HumanKinetics.com**
Email: info@hkcanada.com

E8106

Tell us what you think!
Human Kinetics would love to hear what we
can do to improve the customer experience.
Use this QR code to take our brief survey.

⎢CONTENTS

PART I Warming Up: Physiology 101

PART II The Science of Training Program Design

PART III Special Considerations

If you plan to read this book, you are likely a strong believer in the benefits of regular physical activity and are interested in learning more about how the body responds to exercise and training. In your quest for knowledge, you should be aware that there are many excellent exercise physiology textbooks to choose from. In fact, Dr. Kenney is the author of one of the best-selling exercise physiology textbooks for undergraduate students, *Physiology of Sport and Exercise, Seventh Edition* (Kenney, Wilmorc, & Costill, 2020).

We decided to write a different kind of exercise physiology textbook, one that emphasizes illustrations over text, because we understand that students and busy sport fitness professionals need quick and easy access to accurate and up-to-date scientific information. This text is intended for a variety of people, from those new to the field who want to learn the fundamentals of exercise physiology to professionals who have taken exercise physiology classes in the past and acquired certifications but need to quickly refresh their memories about the scientific underpinnings of exercise and sport.

This book provides an easy, straightforward way for you to review the basic principles of exercise physiology and learn something new that you can put to immediate use. It will also help you refine or design training programs and educate others about the ability of the human body to respond and adapt to regular physical activity. Whether the goal of exercise is to lose weight or gain strength, speed, or stamina, understanding how the body responds physiologically to the stress of exercise should be basic knowledge for all fitness professionals.

Organization of the Book

Practical Guide to Exercise Physiology is divided into three parts. Part I covers how the muscles, heart, lungs, and nervous system respond to exercise and training; how food and drink are converted to fuel; how oxygen enables the breakdown of food into fuel; and how fatigue limits the capacity for exercise yet serves as an important signal to promote the adaptations required for improved fitness and health.

Part II focuses on the design of training programs by reviewing the five principles that should be the basis of every training plan and then highlighting specific design features tailored to increase mass and strength, enhance weight loss, improve speed and power, and maximize aerobic endurance.

Part III is devoted to special considerations such as training clients and athletes to withstand the rigors of heat, cold, and altitude. Also covered are science-based guidelines related to designing effective training programs for children, pregnant women, and older adults.

Special Features

In addition to the numerous photos and detailed illustrations, this second edition of *Practical Guide to Exercise Physiology* contains special features to make science come alive in practical form:

- Scientific terms and concepts are defined and explained using everyday language.
- New content based on recent research has been added, as has a separate chapter on training older adults.
- Numerous examples help you apply sport and nutrition science as you guide clients and athletes to meet their goals.
- Updated artwork and photos are integrated with the content to provide an engaging, highly visual reading experience.
- Sidebars highlight important topics and common questions in exercise physiology.
- Performance Nutrition Spotlight features in each chapter provide the latest advice about how nutrition can be used to support adaptation and improve performance.
- Fun facts add interest throughout the text.
- At the end of each chapter, summary statements and review questions help highlight important information.
- The Index of Common Questions From Clients is a quick reference to help you prepare for inevitable questions.

If you have little background in exercise science, *Practical Guide to Exercise Physiology* gets you started on your sport science journey. And if you have taken classes in exercise physiology, this text will quickly refresh your memory about the fundamental concepts and practical applications of the science related to human physiology, metabolism, and nutrition. We hope the information in this book makes that science come alive in understandable and useful ways.

Ancillaries

One of the key benefits of this new edition is the instructor ancillaries, which include an instructor guide with lecture aids, teachings tips, student assignments, and review questions for each chapter; a large test bank of multiple choice, true-or-false, and fill-in-the-blank questions; and an image bank with all of the figures and tables from the text. Ancillary products supporting this text are free to adopting instructors. Contact your Sales Manager for details about how to access HKPropel, our ancillary delivery and learning platform.

Writing a book is in large part an exercise in teamwork. While the authors spend long hours compiling, collating, reading, distilling, and cross-referencing the needed resources before even beginning to write content, a team of professionals on the publishing end spearheads the behind-the-scenes work required to shepherd the book from its genesis as a simple idea through the many steps required to produce and market the final product. With that backdrop in mind, we would like to thank Amy Tocco and the staff at Human Kinetics for helping bring the second edition of *Practical Guide to Exercise Physiology* to life.

We also appreciate the support and understanding of our wives, both of whom now know all too well what to expect in terms of the occasional grumpiness we might exhibit in trying to meet submission deadlines. And we certainly appreciate all the work Linda and Patti do in helping to make sure we have the time and flexibility required to write a book.

Bob Murray
W. Larry Kenney

Chapter 1

Chapter opening photo: FatCamera/E+/Getty Images
Man doing weightlifting squat, p. 5: Erik Isakson/Getty Images
Man doing deadlift, p. 9: HadelProductions/E+/Getty Images
Soccer player experiencing muscle cramp, p. 12: Nigel French – EMPICS/PA Photos/ Getty Images
Kettlebell weight class, p. 15: Alvarez/E+/Getty Images
Man jogging on treadmill, p. 16: ferrantraite/Getty Images
Participant in a cycling class, p. 17: FatCamera/E+/Getty Images
Woman in weight lifting class, p. 19: MaxRiesgo/iStock/Getty Images
Woman doing lunge with dumbbell, p. 21: Erik Isakson/Getty Images
Woman lifting dumbbells on weight bench, p. 22: Fuse/Corbis/Getty Images

Chapter 2

Chapter opening photo: tacojim/E+/Getty Images
Bread, p. 30: © diegofrias/iStock.com
Bacon, p. 30: © Nirad/iStock.com
Steak, p. 30: © Alex Kladoff/iStock.com
Bananas, p. 41: PhotoDisc
Coffee beans, p. 42: PhotoDisc
Young men at soccer practice, p. 46: Paul Bradbury/Caiaimage/Getty Images
Woman drinking water, p. 48: Vgajic/E+/Getty Images
Firefighter in the heat, p. 49: kali9/E+/Getty Images
Couple drinking water while hiking, p. 50: AVAVA/fotolia.com

Chapter 3

Chapter opening photo: Technotr/iStock/Getty Images
Woman texting on couch, p. 59: Tara Moore/Stone/Getty Images
Exercise class, p. 59: Andres Rodriguez/fotolia.com
Swimmer, p. 59: Corey Jenkins/Image Source/Getty Images
Speed skater, p. 64: John P Kelly/Stone/Getty Images

Chapter 4

Chapter opening photo: Artiga Photo/Corbis/Getty Images
Male sprinters, p. 71: Pete Saloutos/Image Source/Getty Images
Fatigued athlete, p. 76: Peathegee Inc/Getty Images
Tired woman in gym, p. 80: golubovy/Getty Images/Getty Images
Weary athlete taking a break, p. 84: Corey Jenkins/Image Source/Getty Images

Chapter 5

Chapter opening photo: Johner Images - Berggren, Hans/Brand X Pictures/Getty Images
Athlete reviewing training plan, p. 92: EmirMemedovski/E+/Getty Images
Woman doing dumbbell curls, p. 93: Stockbyte/Corbis
Woman doing dumbbell press, p. 95: Vitapix/E+/Getty Images
Male cross country skier, p. 95: John P Kelly/Stone/Getty Images
Man running in the park, p. 97: Georgijevic/iStock/Getty Images
Woman on training run, p. 100: Svetikd/E+/Getty Images
Fatigued tennis player, p. 104: Tim Clayton - Corbis/Getty Images

Chapter 6

Chapter opening photo: MRBIG_PHOTOGRAPHY/E+/Getty Images
Male gymnast on rings, p. 111: Fuse/Corbis/Getty Images
Woman doing squats with medicine ball, p. 113: yoh4nn/E+/Getty Images
Electrical muscle simulation device, p. 123: YOSHIKAZU TSUNO/AFP via Getty Images
Chicken, p. 124: pada smith/iStock/Getty Images
Eggs, p. 124: Milanfoto/E+/Getty Images

Chapter 7

Chapter opening photo: Laflor/E+/Getty Images
Woman reading in front of fire, p. 131: Westend61/Getty Images
Biker snacking, p. 136: Fancy/Veer/Corbis/Getty Images
Woman doing crunches, p. 140: Photodisc/Getty Images

Chapter 8

Chapter opening photo: David Madison/Stone/Getty Images
Woman hurdling, p. 149: RyanJLane/E+/Getty Images
Javelin throw, p. 150: © Becky Miller/Gopher Track Shots
Female softball player, p. 152: EHStock/iStock/Getty Images
Man running up stairs, p. 154: Westend61/Getty Images
Man jumping rope, p. 158: Skynesher/E+

Chapter 9

Chapter opening photo: Per Breiehagen/Stone
Woman testing for $\dot{V}O_{2\,Max}$, p. 164: technotr/iStockphoto/Getty Images
Ultra-marathoners, p. 167: JEAN-PHILIPPE KSIAZEK/AFP via Getty Images
Female soccer player, p. 168: Corey Jenkins/Image Source/Getty Images
Eliud Kipchoge, p. 169: HERBERT NEUBAUER/APA/AFP via Getty Images
Mountain bikers, p. 170: Ascent Xmedia/Stone/Getty Images
Female swimmer, p. 173: Corey Jenkins/Image Source
Woman using battle ropes, p. 176: Sushiman/iStock/Getty Images
Fatigued female biker, p. 178: Klaus Vedfelt/DigitalVision/Getty Images

Chapter 10

Chapter opening photo: Westend61/Getty Images
Fatigued man drinking water, p. 189: laflor/Getty Images
Woman running in mountains, p. 196: Miljko/E+/Getty Images

Chapter 11

Chapter opening photo: Thomas Barwick/Stone/Getty Images
Girl's basketball team, p. 203: Brand X Pictures
Young athlete snacking, p. 204: Lite Productions/Getty Images
Child doing weightlifting squat, p. 205: SDI Productions/E+/Getty Images
Children running in gym, p. 206: FatCamera/E+/Getty Images
Female gymnast on balance beam, p. 208: M_a_y_a/E+/Getty Images
Pregnant woman jogging, p. 210: Jose Luis Pelaez Inc/DigitalVision/Getty Images

Chapter 12

Chapter opening photo: Adamkaz/E+/Getty Images
Man running up stairs, p. 218: MStudioImages/E+/Getty Images
Man and woman jogging on the beach, p. 220: Eyewire
Woman lifting dumbbells, p. 221: Jose Luis Pelaez Inc/DigitalVision

PART I

Warming Up: Physiology 101

CHAPTER ONE

Muscles Move Us

Objectives

- Understand the basics of how muscles function.
- Learn how muscles respond to exercise and adapt to training.
- Discover the role of genetics in training and performance.

Exercise physiology is the study of how the body responds to exercise and adapts to physical training, so what better place to start this book than with skeletal muscle cells, the microscopic engines whose coordinated efforts convert chemical power into motion? During physical activity, your muscles take center stage. While you're also aware that heart rate has increased and breathing becomes heavier, it's natural that you're most tuned in to your muscles. After all, one of the goals of exercise training is to change muscles: to make them stronger, quicker to respond, more powerful, and more resistant to fatigue. With proper training, improvements in all aspects of muscle function are possible. But muscles cannot function in isolation, and as you train your muscles, you're also training your nervous system, heart, lungs, blood vessels, liver, kidneys, and many other organs and tissues. Planning an effective training program requires keeping in mind that big picture—a picture that involves more than just muscles.

But because muscle is the foundation for all movement, a review of basic muscle physiology is a great place to start.

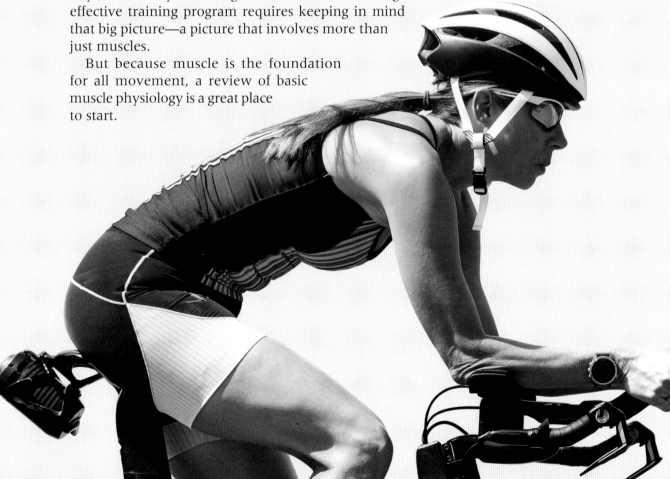

How Do Muscles Work?

Take a quick look at figure 1.1. Similar figures appear in many textbooks because certain basic parts of skeletal muscle are important to recognize. When talking about muscles, you most likely think of skeletal muscle because that is the type of muscle that is involved in exercise and that you feel working and tiring and aching. But cardiac muscle in the heart and smooth muscle in blood vessels and the gastrointestinal tract are also very much involved in supporting the body's ability to exercise. Cardiac muscle cells and smooth muscle cells are structured differently compared to skeletal muscle cells, yet the job of all three types of muscle cells is to contract and relax. For now, we will focus on skeletal muscle, the type of muscle that moves your body.

When a motor nerve is stimulated, all the muscle cells it innervates contract in unison.

▌FIGURE 1.1 The structure of muscle.

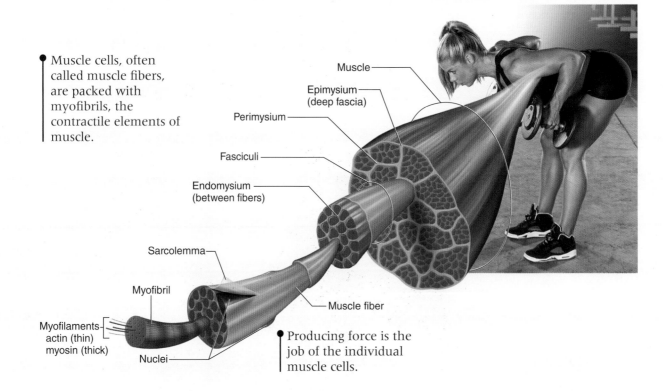

Muscle cells, often called muscle fibers, are packed with myofibrils, the contractile elements of muscle.

Muscle
Epimysium (deep fascia)
Perimysium
Fasciculi
Endomysium (between fibers)
Sarcolemma
Myofibril
Myofilaments—actin (thin) myosin (thick)
Nuclei
Muscle fiber

Producing force is the job of the individual muscle cells.

Even though skeletal muscles come in many shapes and sizes, they all share a common internal structure. Skeletal muscles are simply bundles (called *fasciculi*) of individual muscle cells arranged in groups (*motor units*) controlled by individual nerves (*alpha motor neurons*; see figure 1.2) so that all the cells in the group contract in unison. Each muscle cell is packed with contractile proteins (the myofibrils *actin* and *myosin*), enzymes (to help speed up reactions), nuclei (for protein production), mitochondria (for energy production), glycogen (the storage form of glucose used by the cell for energy), and sarcoplasmic reticulum (to aid contraction and relaxation; see figure 1.4). The structure of each cell is supported on the inside by a framework of proteins and on the outside by various types of connective tissues that support individual cells, bundles of cells, and the entire muscle. The terms *endomysium*, *perimysium*, and *epimysium* refer to these connective tissues.

The basic job of muscle is to move bones around their joints. This requires muscles to contract with enough force to get that job done, whether that entails lifting a heavy weight just once, sprinting a short distance, or cycling a long distance.

The Electrical Connection

Skeletal muscle fibers don't contract on their own but usually require nerve input from the brain (though some fast reflex movements involve only spinal nerves and muscles). Figure 1.2 is a simple illustration of one nerve (a motor neuron) connected to three muscle cells. The motor neuron and its attached muscle cells are referred to as a *motor unit*. A single motor neuron may be connected to (may innervate) dozens, hundreds, or even thousands of individual muscle cells, depending on the size and function of the muscle. When the motor neuron fires, all the muscle cells in that motor unit contract in unison. For movements that require little strength, such as picking up a fork, only a few motor units are activated. For movements that require maximal strength, a maximal number of available motor units are activated and those motor units are rapidly stimulated, a response known as *rate coding*. When an untrained person begins strength training, most of the initial

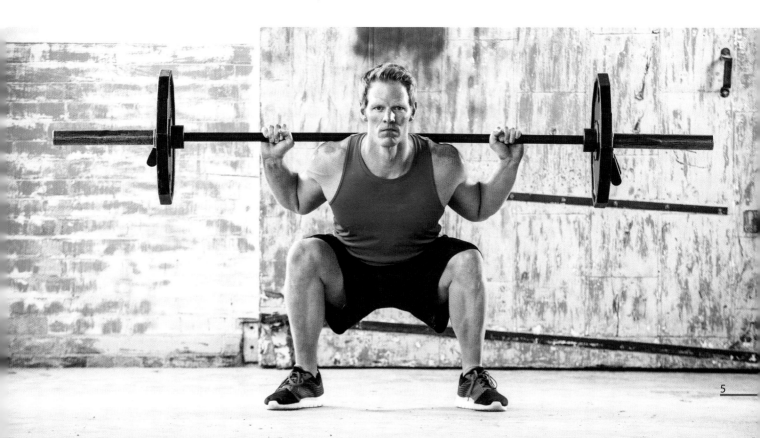

improvement in muscle strength over the first couple months is due to increased recruitment of motor units by the central nervous system, a good example of how muscles operate in cooperation with other organ systems.

The order in which motor units are activated depends in part upon the size of the nerve and its conduction velocity. In every movement—including all-out efforts—slow motor units are recruited first to get things moving. Faster contraction speeds actually mean less force production because fewer myosin cross bridges have time to attach to actin filaments. This inverse relationship between the speed of muscle contraction and force production is referred to as the *force-velocity curve*. (Myosin is considered a *motor protein* because the heads of the myosin cross-bridge molecules that attach to actin filaments operate like tiny motors to pull actin toward the center of the sarcomere. Cells contain many different types of motor proteins that aid in the movement of molecules from one part of the cell to another.)

It's important to understand how nerves cause muscles to contract because if that process is disrupted, strength is impaired and cramps can occur, as detailed in chapter 4. Figure 1.3 is a simple overview of the various steps required for muscle to contract, which will give you a basic understanding (or review) of how skeletal muscle cells contract.

Some alpha motor neurons can be more than 3 feet (about 1 m) long.

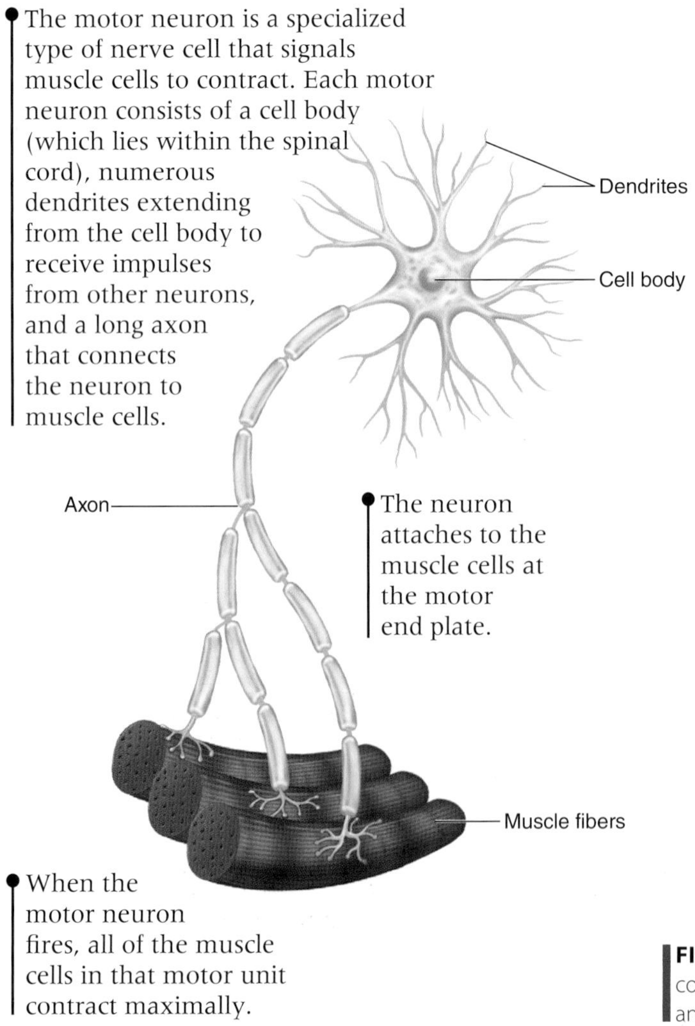

The motor neuron is a specialized type of nerve cell that signals muscle cells to contract. Each motor neuron consists of a cell body (which lies within the spinal cord), numerous dendrites extending from the cell body to receive impulses from other neurons, and a long axon that connects the neuron to muscle cells.

Dendrites

Cell body

Axon

The neuron attaches to the muscle cells at the motor end plate.

Muscle fibers

When the motor neuron fires, all of the muscle cells in that motor unit contract maximally.

FIGURE 1.2 A motor unit, consisting of a motor neuron and the fibers it innervates.

▌FIGURE 1.3 The series of events that cause muscle cells to contract.

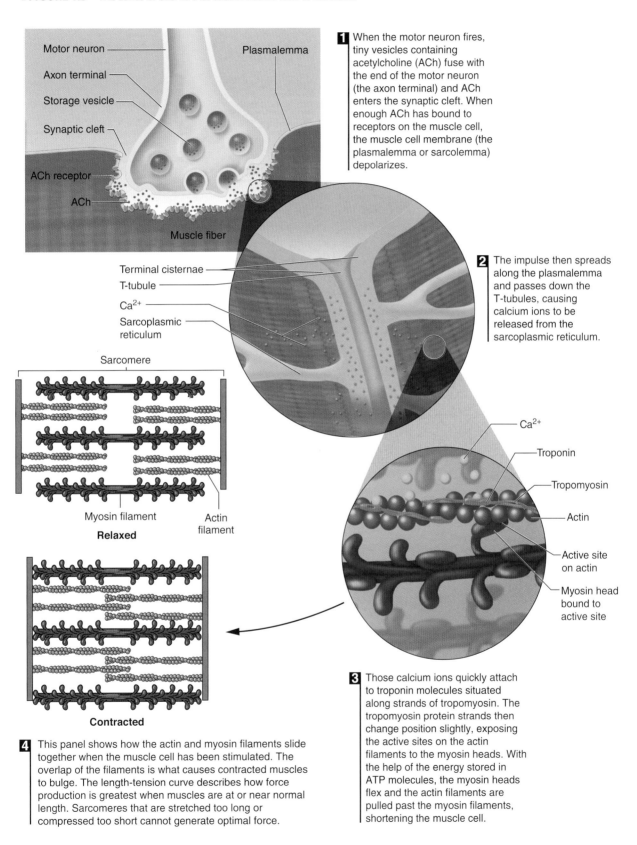

1 When the motor neuron fires, tiny vesicles containing acetylcholine (ACh) fuse with the end of the motor neuron (the axon terminal) and ACh enters the synaptic cleft. When enough ACh has bound to receptors on the muscle cell, the muscle cell membrane (the plasmalemma or sarcolemma) depolarizes.

Motor neuron — Plasmalemma
Axon terminal
Storage vesicle
Synaptic cleft
ACh receptor
ACh
Muscle fiber

Terminal cisternae
T-tubule
Ca^{2+}
Sarcoplasmic reticulum

2 The impulse then spreads along the plasmalemma and passes down the T-tubules, causing calcium ions to be released from the sarcoplasmic reticulum.

Ca^{2+}
Troponin
Tropomyosin
Actin
Active site on actin
Myosin head bound to active site

Sarcomere

Myosin filament   Actin filament
Relaxed

Contracted

4 This panel shows how the actin and myosin filaments slide together when the muscle cell has been stimulated. The overlap of the filaments is what causes contracted muscles to bulge. The length-tension curve describes how force production is greatest when muscles are at or near normal length. Sarcomeres that are stretched too long or compressed too short cannot generate optimal force.

3 Those calcium ions quickly attach to troponin molecules situated along strands of tropomyosin. The tropomyosin protein strands then change position slightly, exposing the active sites on the actin filaments to the myosin heads. With the help of the energy stored in ATP molecules, the myosin heads flex and the actin filaments are pulled past the myosin filaments, shortening the muscle cell.

Here is the short version of how a muscle contracts:

If you decide to do a biceps curl with a heavy weight, nerve impulses travel from the brain to the spine and from the spine down motor neurons to the biceps muscle cells within those motor units. When the impulses reach the junctions between the motor neuron and each muscle cell (called the *neuromuscular junction*), a *neurotransmitter* called *acetylcholine* is released into the space between the nerve and the muscle (that space is called the *synapse* or the synaptic cleft). The impulses are thereby transmitted from the motor neuron to all the muscle cells it innervates, causing those cells to contract in unison. But before the cells contract, the impulses have to first travel across the entire muscle cell membrane (the sarcolemma or plasmalemma), dipping instantaneously into the interior of each cell through T-tubules (*transverse tubules*). Each impulse causes calcium ions (calcium molecules) to be released from the *sarcoplasmic reticulum*; this release of calcium ions causes actin and myosin filaments to interact in a way that causes muscle to contract (see figure 1.3 for more detail about the *sliding-filament theory* of muscle contraction). When the nerve impulses stop, the calcium ions are instantly taken back into the sarcoplasmic reticulum and the muscle cells relax.

Figure 1.4 shows how the plasmalemma (sarcolemma) is connected to the T-tubules and how the sarcoplasmic reticulum (SR) surrounds the myofibrils within a single muscle

Myosin is just one of many motor proteins.

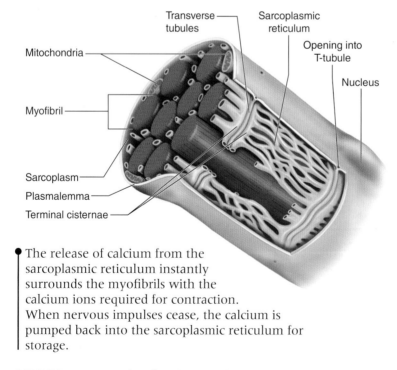

Transverse tubules · Sarcoplasmic reticulum · Opening into T-tubule · Nucleus · Mitochondria · Myofibril · Sarcoplasm · Plasmalemma · Terminal cisternae

The release of calcium from the sarcoplasmic reticulum instantly surrounds the myofibrils with the calcium ions required for contraction. When nervous impulses cease, the calcium is pumped back into the sarcoplasmic reticulum for storage.

FIGURE 1.4 A muscle cell is a very crowded space. Everything about the cell supports muscle contractions, from single, all-out, maximal-strength contractions to the repeated contractions needed for sustaining endurance activities.

cell. Jammed into the packed space inside muscle cells are a variety of enzymes needed for energy (ATP) production, glycogen molecules (the storage form of glucose), fat molecules, and many other molecules and structures.

One of those other molecules is the protein titin. In recent years, scientists have learned that titin not only aids in maintaining the overall structure of the muscle fiber, keeping the sliding filaments (actin and myosin) in line, but also is important in muscle strength, particularly as muscle lengthens (eccentric contractions), with titin acting as a molecular spring. It seems that calcium ions cause titin to stiffen, helping to explain why muscles are so much stronger during eccentric (lengthening) contractions than during concentric (shortening) contractions. It may be that muscle cells actually contain three contractile proteins: actin, myosin, and titin.

Titin is the largest known protein, consisting of 34,350 amino acids. As a result, the formal chemical name for titin contains 189,819 letters and takes more than 3 hours to pronounce, making it the longest word in the English language.

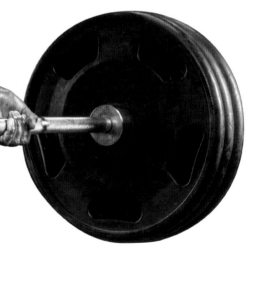

Key Terms for Muscle Contraction

Concentric contraction—Force is produced as the muscle shortens, as in raising a weight.

Eccentric contraction—Force is produced as the muscle lengthens, as in lowering a weight.

Isometric contraction—Force is produced with no change in muscle length, as in pushing against a wall.

Different Cell Types for Different Jobs

Not surprisingly, different types of muscle cells enable humans to perform explosive movements of short duration as well as complete amazing feats of endurance exercise. The muscle fiber (cell) types are simply referred to as type I (slow-twitch) and type II (fast-twitch). Type I fibers are better suited for endurance exercise and type II fibers are better suited for sprints or other brief, powerful movements. Figure 1.5 shows a cross-section of muscle stained to show the different fiber types. Interestingly, motor units contain only one fiber type. The motor neurons that innervate type I motor units are smaller in diameter than the neurons that supply type II motor units. In addition to that difference, type I motor units contain fewer fibers than type II motor units. As a result, type II motor units develop more force when they are activated.

A basic concept in muscle physiology is that small motor units are recruited before larger motor units. The official name for this concept is *Henneman's size principle*, named after Elwood Henneman, the American scientist who is credited with describing the concept in the 1960s. Regardless of the intensity of the effort, smaller type I motor units are recruited before larger type II motor units. In other words, even during all-out sprints or explosive movements such as jumping or Olympic weightlifting, a mix of motor units helps accomplish those tasks.

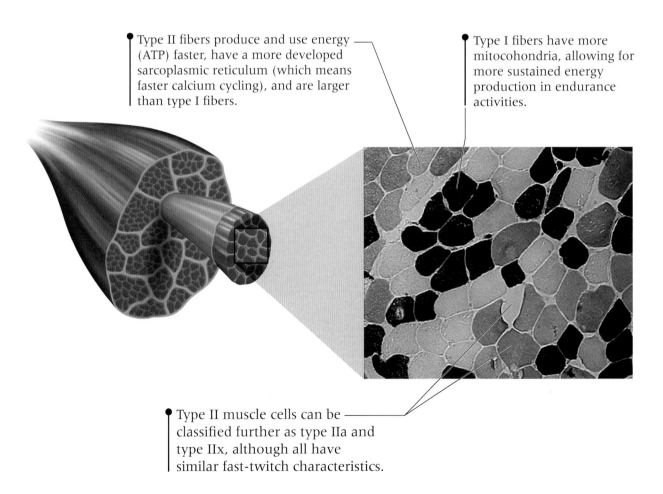

Type II fibers produce and use energy (ATP) faster, have a more developed sarcoplasmic reticulum (which means faster calcium cycling), and are larger than type I fibers.

Type I fibers have more mitocohondria, allowing for more sustained energy production in endurance activities.

Type II muscle cells can be classified further as type IIa and type IIx, although all have similar fast-twitch characteristics.

FIGURE 1.5 Muscle cells are called on to accomplish all sorts of tasks, so it should be no surprise that cells are specialized for distinct functions.

Micrograph reprinted from W.L. Kenney, J. H. Wilmore, and D.L. Costill, 2020, *Physiology of Sport and Exercise,* 7th ed. (Champaign, IL: Human Kinetics), 41. By permission of D.L. Costill.

Most muscles are roughly 50% fast-twitch (type II) and 50% slow-twitch (type I), but these proportions can vary widely, as shown in table 1.1. Some elite distance runners have leg muscles in which over 90% of the muscle cells are slow-twitch (type I) fibers, while some elite sprinters have the opposite mix. Although the ratio of fiber types is determined by genetics, proper training can improve the function of any muscle cell—the very basis for greater fitness and performance.

Arms and legs contain a similar proportion of type I and type II muscle cells, although those proportions vary from person to person.

TABLE 1.1   **Percentages of Type I and Type II Fibers in Muscles of Male and Female Athletes**

Sport	Sex	Muscle	% type I	% type II
Sprint runners	M	Gastrocnemius	24	76
	F	Gastrocnemius	27	73
Distance runners	M	Gastrocnemius	79	21
	F	Gastrocnemius	69	31
Cyclists	M	Vastus lateralis	57	43
	F	Vastus lateralis	51	49
Swimmers	M	Posterior deltoid	67	33
Weightlifters	M	Gastrocnemius	44	56
	M	Deltoid	53	47
Triathletes	M	Posterior deltoid	60	40
	M	Vastus lateralis	63	37
	M	Gastrocnemius	59	41
Canoeists	M	Posterior deltoid	71	29
Shot-putters	M	Gastrocnemius	38	62
Nonathletes	M	Vastus lateralis	47	53
	F	Gastrocnemius	52	48

Adapted by permission from W.L. Kenney, J.H. Wilmore, and D.L. Costill, *Physiology of Sport and Exercise*, 7th ed. (Champaign, IL: Human Kinetics, 2020), 47.

What Happens When Muscles Stretch?

Why do muscles feel tight whenever they are stretched? For example, when you try to touch your toes while the knees are locked, the hamstring muscles stretch and you feel that tension. But what causes the tension? For many decades, the prevailing theory was that the passive tension produced when a muscle is stretched was due to an increased tension in the connective tissues surrounding the muscles. It turns out those connective tissues may not be responsible for the forces produced when a muscle is stretched. Eccentric muscle contractions stretch muscle cells, reducing the opportunity for actin and myosin to interact. Yet eccentric contractions are very powerful. Recent research has shown that the structural protein titin plays an important role in force production during eccentric contractions. Titin is an enormous protein that acts like a spring inside each skeletal muscle cell. Stretch any muscle and the titin molecules within the muscle cells are also stretched. Just as a rubber band increases its tension when stretched, so does titin, adding to the force produced by actin and myosin. In that regard, titin may be considered the third contractile protein in muscle cells.

You've had muscle cramps of one sort or another. Usually those cramps amount to little more than a temporary nuisance or, at worst, cause you to stop exercising for the day. Muscle cramps are a good example of how muscle function is integrated with central nervous system activity and nutrition.

Let's start with three things that scientists know about muscle cramps: (1) not all muscle cramps are the same; (2) there is no single cause for muscle cramps; and (3) for those reasons, there is no one way to prevent muscle cramping.

The most common muscle cramp occurs when a single muscle group contracts and remains contracted, causing immediate, localized pain. Examples are cramped calf muscles in runners or cyclists, cramped hamstrings in football players, cramped muscles in the feet of swimmers, and cramped leg muscles during sleep, usually in older adults.

Some cramps appear to be caused by an overstimulation of nerve input to muscles. Others likely occur from dehydration or a combination of dehydration and salt loss in sweat. The cramps that some swimmers have in their feet appear to be caused by local fatigue resulting from keeping their feet pointed while they swim. The cramping that can occur during sleep and other nonexercise occasions may be due to nerve–muscle imbalance (more about that in a bit). Whole-body muscle cramps—sometimes called "heat cramps," the worst of all cramping—are thought to result from severe dehydration and salt loss during high-intensity or prolonged exercise.

The very nature of a muscle cramp indicates that there is an imbalance in the normal interaction between the motor nerve and the muscle. Muscles usually contract only in response to nerve input, so a sustained cramp is evidence of sustained, abnormal input from the nerves supplying that muscle.

In 1878, doctors noticed that gold miners in Nevada were prone to whole-body muscle cramps. The same was true of workers on the Hoover Dam and coal shovelers in the engine rooms on steam ships. In all cases, the cramps were prevented when the workers increased their fluid and salt intake. Staying well hydrated, well fueled (with carbohydrate), and well salted (with electrolytes) prevents the muscle cramping associated with dehydration, fatigue, and salt loss.

Once cramps hit, there is little to do but to stop exercise and stretch (or be stretched). Severe, whole-body muscle cramps often require intravenous saline infusion and a prescription muscle relaxant. Other cramp remedies include drinking a small volume of pickle juice or spices such as capsaicin, ginger, and cinnamon; taking a taste of mustard; eating bananas or oranges; and receiving injections of calcium gluconate or magnesium sulfate. Of all those remedies, only pickle juice and the spice mixture have some scientific evidence to support their use. Researchers think that the acetic acid (vinegar) in pickle juice and the spice mixture stimulate receptors in the mouth, throat, and esophagus that help reduce the nerve input to cramped muscles by way of a mouth-brain-muscle connection.

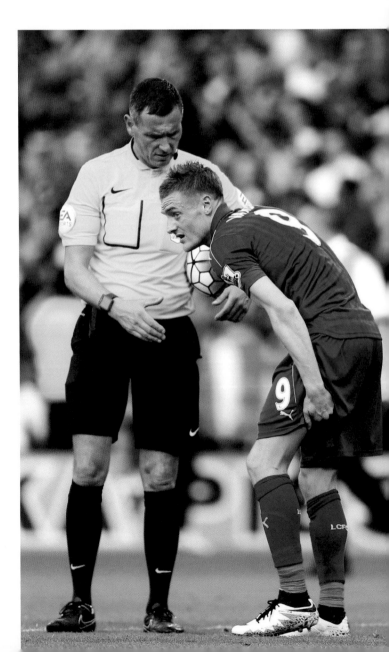

What Determines Competitive Success?

Why do some people excel at sports and others struggle? Look at any team in any sport and you'll find a range of fitness levels, sport skills, and competitive success, even though the team members are all exposed to similar training. So why is it that a similar stimulus results in various degrees of adaptation? Figure 1.6 provides some insights and reflects important aspects of the content of this book.

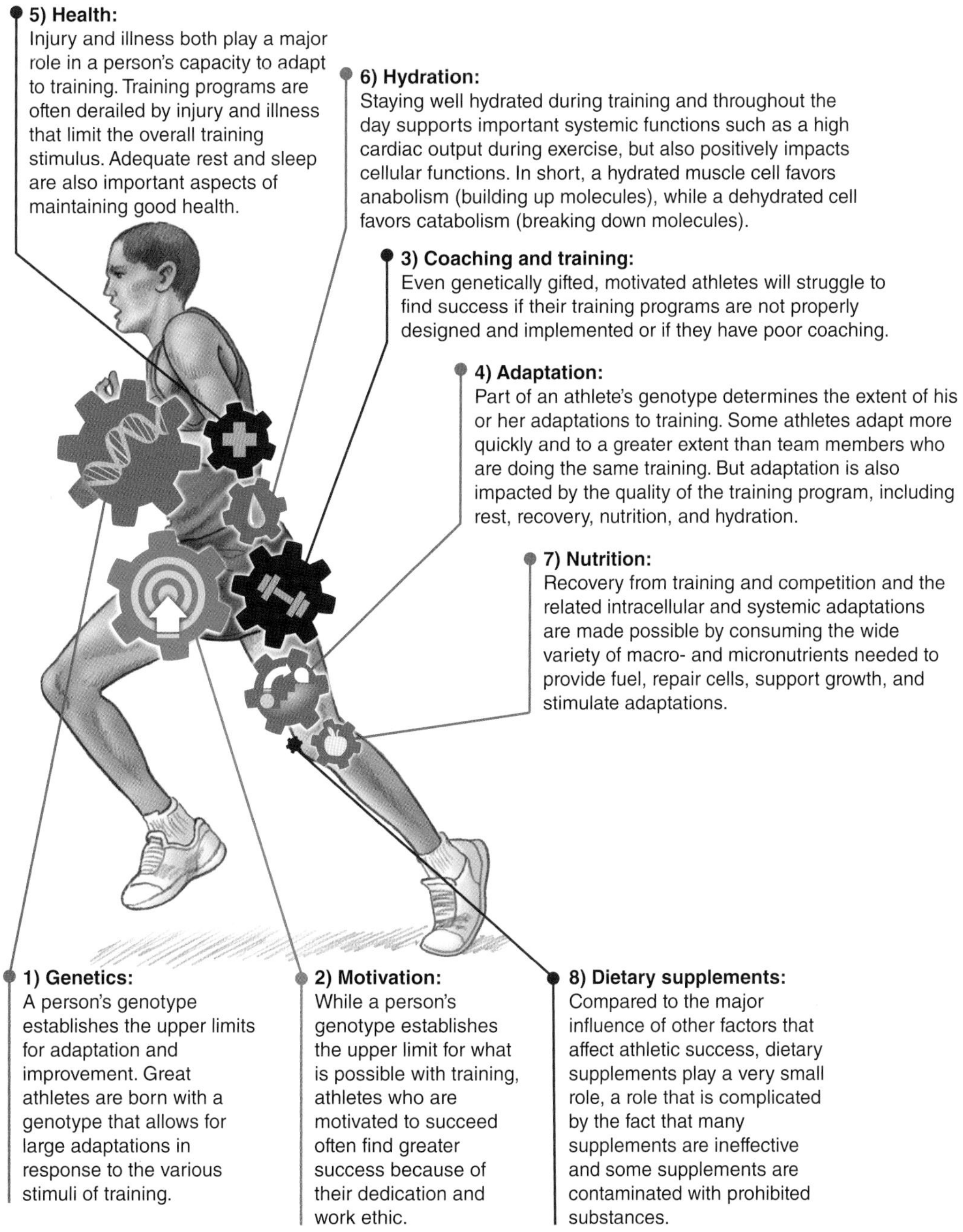

5) Health:
Injury and illness both play a major role in a person's capacity to adapt to training. Training programs are often derailed by injury and illness that limit the overall training stimulus. Adequate rest and sleep are also important aspects of maintaining good health.

6) Hydration:
Staying well hydrated during training and throughout the day supports important systemic functions such as a high cardiac output during exercise, but also positively impacts cellular functions. In short, a hydrated muscle cell favors anabolism (building up molecules), while a dehydrated cell favors catabolism (breaking down molecules).

3) Coaching and training:
Even genetically gifted, motivated athletes will struggle to find success if their training programs are not properly designed and implemented or if they have poor coaching.

4) Adaptation:
Part of an athlete's genotype determines the extent of his or her adaptations to training. Some athletes adapt more quickly and to a greater extent than team members who are doing the same training. But adaptation is also impacted by the quality of the training program, including rest, recovery, nutrition, and hydration.

7) Nutrition:
Recovery from training and competition and the related intracellular and systemic adaptations are made possible by consuming the wide variety of macro- and micronutrients needed to provide fuel, repair cells, support growth, and stimulate adaptations.

1) Genetics:
A person's genotype establishes the upper limits for adaptation and improvement. Great athletes are born with a genotype that allows for large adaptations in response to the various stimuli of training.

2) Motivation:
While a person's genotype establishes the upper limit for what is possible with training, athletes who are motivated to succeed often find greater success because of their dedication and work ethic.

8) Dietary supplements:
Compared to the major influence of other factors that affect athletic success, dietary supplements play a very small role, a role that is complicated by the fact that many supplements are ineffective and some supplements are contaminated with prohibited substances.

Figure 1.6   Many factors affect a person's success in sport. Some are within the athlete's control and others are not.

Thanks to Dr. Ronald J. Maughan, St. Andrews University, Scotland, for the initial concept that inspired this figure.

How Do Muscles Adapt to Training?

In the simplest terms, when muscles are stressed by exercise, they gradually increase their capacity to handle that stress. For instance, muscles adapt to strength training by increasing the number of motor units that are recruited during weightlifting and by producing more myofibrillar proteins (actin, myosin, and other proteins involved in muscle contraction). Those changes result in increased strength and often increased muscle size. With endurance training, muscles adapt by increasing the number and size of energy-producing mitochondria as well as the enzymes used to break down glycogen, glucose, and fatty acids for energy.

All these adaptations occur because regular training results in changes in the many nuclei contained in each muscle cell. The DNA in the nucleus of every muscle cell contains genes that are the blueprints for every protein within a muscle cell, such as contractile proteins, structural proteins, regulatory proteins, mitochondrial proteins, motor proteins, and enzymes. With training, changes in gene expression in the cell lead to increased production of functional proteins.

As depicted in figure 1.7, the stimulus of training eventually results in the desired responses. Those adaptations are made possible by a variety of facilitators. For example, the response to training will be less than optimal if the client or athlete is often dehydrated, eats poorly, and doesn't get enough rest. Optimal responses to training are made possible by adaptations in the nervous, immune, and hormonal (*endocrine*) systems, all of which are disrupted by poor hydration, nutrition, and rest. In other words, for optimal responses to occur, a great training program has to be complemented by proper hydration, nutrition, and rest.

Skeletal muscles are roughly 75% water. In other words, if you gain 10 pounds of muscle, you actually gain 7.5 pounds of water and 2.5 pounds of contractile proteins and other cellular components.

▌FIGURE 1.7 Muscle cells adapt to the stress of training in ways that improve the muscle's capacity for exercise.

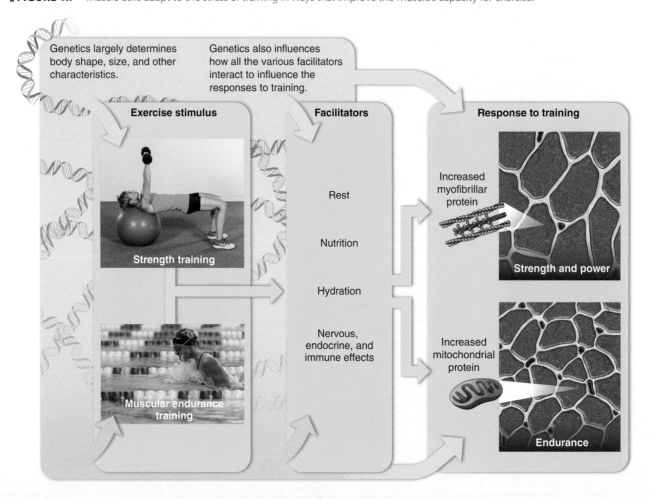

Genetics largely determines body shape, size, and other characteristics.

Genetics also influences how all the various facilitators interact to influence the responses to training.

Exercise stimulus

Strength training

Muscular endurance training

Facilitators

Rest

Nutrition

Hydration

Nervous, endocrine, and immune effects

Response to training

Increased myofibrillar protein

Strength and power

Increased mitochondrial protein

Endurance

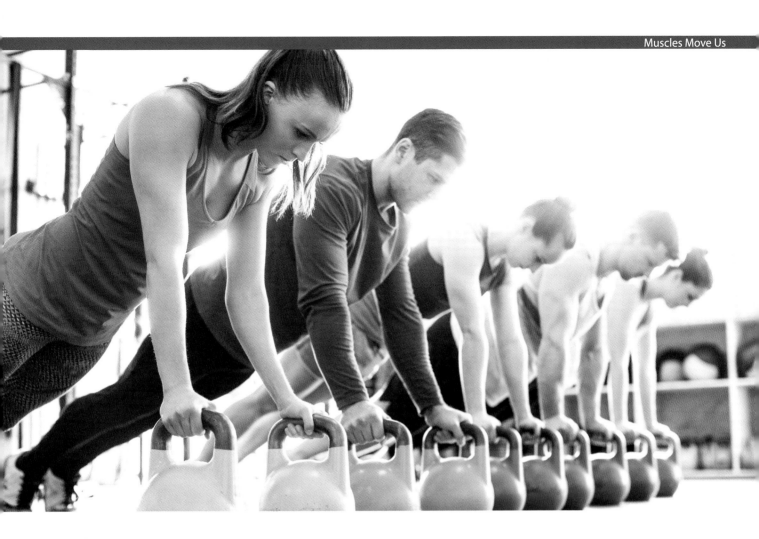

Genetics also plays a large role in the adaptations that result from training. Everyone adapts uniquely to exercise training because everyone has a unique genetic makeup. Your genes help determine the speed and magnitude of your response to training. Even if every athlete or client began a training program with exactly the same strength and fitness characteristics, some would adapt to the training faster than others, making greater gains in strength, speed, and endurance. In other words, some people are *high responders* and some are *low responders*. Sex also plays a role in the capacity for adaptations to training. For example, men's muscles typically experience more hypertrophy as a result of strength training because of the greater testosterone levels in men. You'll learn more about these differences later in this book.

Genetics plays a role in adaptation to training because your genetic makeup determines the upper limits of strength, speed, and endurance. For example, research has shown that 25% to 50% of the improvement in maximal oxygen uptake ($\dot{V}O_{2max}$) is determined by genetics. The painful truth is that no matter how hard some people train, the highest $\dot{V}O_{2max}$ they may be able to attain might be lower than that of an untrained individual who has the genetic predisposition for a high $\dot{V}O_{2max}$. The same is true for strength, speed, agility, flexibility, and other athletic characteristics.

If genes determine only part of the ability to adapt to training, what determines the other part? That's where work ethic, dedication, rest, nutrition, and hydration enter the picture. The adaptations that result from exercise training require months of consistent hard work. That regular overload on muscle cells, combined with adequate rest, proper hydration, and ample nutrition, creates and supports the intracellular environment that optimizes the production of all the functional proteins that are needed for increased strength, speed, and stamina.

> **Genetics determines the upper limits for strength, speed, power, and endurance.**

Adaptations to Aerobic, Anaerobic, and Strength Training

Muscle contractions move the body, and muscle cell mitochondria are the organelles that supply much of the energy for the contractions. The muscle cell engines, like all engines, have to be fueled and cooled, and waste products have to be removed. Those jobs fall to the lungs, heart, vasculature, liver, and kidneys with the help of endocrine glands (such as the pituitary, hypothalamus, thyroid,

Adaptations to Aerobic Training

In the Heart

- Increased size of the heart (cardiac hypertrophy)
- Increased thickness of the heart's left ventricle
- Reduced resting heart rate
- Faster recovery of heart rate after exercise bouts
- Increased stroke volume (the volume of blood per heartbeat)
- Increased maximal cardiac output (the volume of blood pumped by the heart each minute)

In the Muscles

- Increased maximal oxygen uptake ($\dot{V}O_{2max}$)
- Increased endurance capacity
- Increased oxygen extraction from the blood by active muscles
- Increased enzymes involved in energy (ATP) production from carbohydrate and fat
- Increased muscle and liver glycogen content
- Increased cross-sectional area of type I muscle cells
- Increased muscle myoglobin content
- Increased number and size of muscle cell mitochondria
- Increased lactate threshold
- Increased maximal lactate production
- Increased reliance on fatty acids for fuel at submaximal intensities

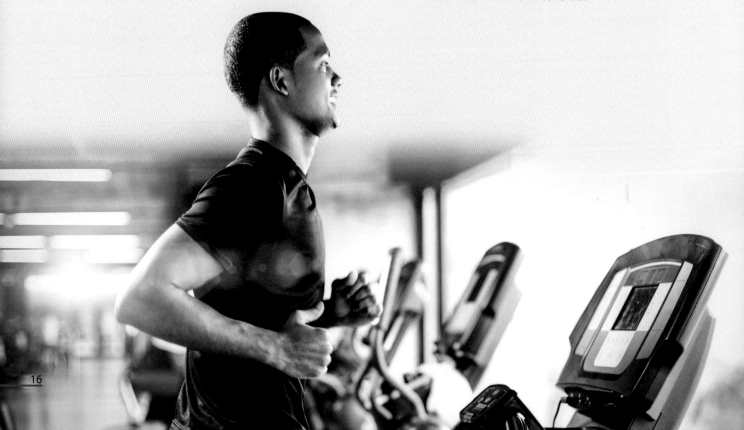

pancreas, and adrenal glands). As muscle cells adapt to training, so do the tissues and organs that support muscle function.

Following is a list of many of the adaptations that result from aerobic (endurance) training, all of which help support the continued contraction of skeletal muscle during endurance exercise. This long list of adaptations is evidence that exercise is powerful stuff when it comes to promoting changes that improve health and performance.

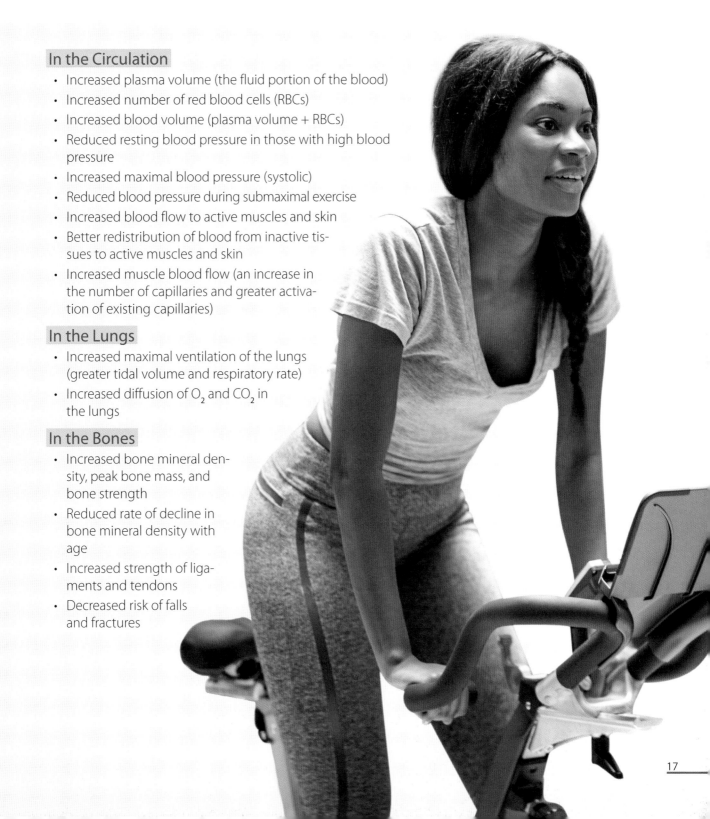

In the Circulation

- Increased plasma volume (the fluid portion of the blood)
- Increased number of red blood cells (RBCs)
- Increased blood volume (plasma volume + RBCs)
- Reduced resting blood pressure in those with high blood pressure
- Increased maximal blood pressure (systolic)
- Reduced blood pressure during submaximal exercise
- Increased blood flow to active muscles and skin
- Better redistribution of blood from inactive tissues to active muscles and skin
- Increased muscle blood flow (an increase in the number of capillaries and greater activation of existing capillaries)

In the Lungs

- Increased maximal ventilation of the lungs (greater tidal volume and respiratory rate)
- Increased diffusion of O_2 and CO_2 in the lungs

In the Bones

- Increased bone mineral density, peak bone mass, and bone strength
- Reduced rate of decline in bone mineral density with age
- Increased strength of ligaments and tendons
- Decreased risk of falls and fractures

Training for sprint and power events in sports

such as running, swimming, soccer, football, basketball, wrestling, volleyball, boxing, hockey, and rugby produces some of the same adaptations as seen with endurance training, but other adaptations occur that are better suited to meet the demands of all-out activities of fairly short duration. This list includes many of the adaptations that occur as a result of anaerobic training programs.

Anaerobic training programs can also be effective at improving aerobic capacity and performance. That's not to say that endurance athletes should switch training programs to emphasize anaerobic training (such as high-intensity interval training; HIIT), but endurance athletes can improve their speed and power without sacrificing their aerobic fitness. Another practical benefit of anaerobic training of fairly short duration (HIIT; for example, a 10-minute warm-up followed by six 30-second sprints separated by 3 minutes of rest) is that improvements in both anaerobic and aerobic capacity can be had with very little investment in

Adaptations to Anaerobic Training
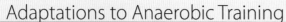
Anaerobic training includes HIIT, or high-intensity interval training.

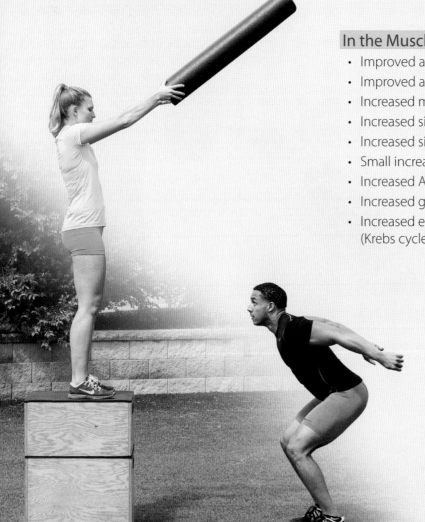

In the Muscles
- Improved anaerobic power and capacity
- Improved aerobic power and capacity
- Increased muscle strength
- Increased size of type II fibers
- Increased size of type I fibers but less so than type II
- Small increase in the percentage of type II fibers
- Increased ATP-PCr enzyme activities
- Increased glycolytic enzyme activities
- Increased enzymes involved in aerobic ATP production (Krebs cycle)

In the Bones
- Increased bone mineral density, peak bone mass, and bone strength
- Reduced rate of decline in bone mineral density with age
- Increased strength of ligaments and tendons
- Decreased risk of falls and fractures

exercise time, a real benefit for anyone who finds it difficult to set aside an hour or two for daily workouts. We revisit this topic in chapter 8.

Strength training produces the kinds of adaptations that you might expect. As mentioned earlier in this chapter, much of the initial gain in strength results from changes in the central nervous system that promote increased recruitment of motor units. Subsequent increases in strength and mass occur over weeks and months as muscles lay down more contractile proteins. Most types of training also benefit bones and ligaments, and that is especially true of activities that involve weight bearing or repeated high impact because such activities place rapid strain on bones, a key trigger for producing stronger bones. Good examples are running, gymnastics, strength training, and power training. Cycling, swimming, and other sports in which there is less stress on bones may actually reduce bone mineral density and bone strength, an additional reason that cross-training can be beneficial.

Adaptations to Strength Training

In the Muscles

- More motor units recruited
- Greater stimulation frequency of motor units
- More synchronous recruiting of motor units
- Reduced inhibition of motor units
- Increased muscle cell size (hypertrophy)
- Possibly a small increase in the number of muscle cells (hyperplasia)

In the Bones

- Increased bone mineral density, peak bone mass, and bone strength
- Reduced rate of decline in bone mineral density with age
- Increased strength of ligaments and tendons
- Decreased risk of falls and fractures

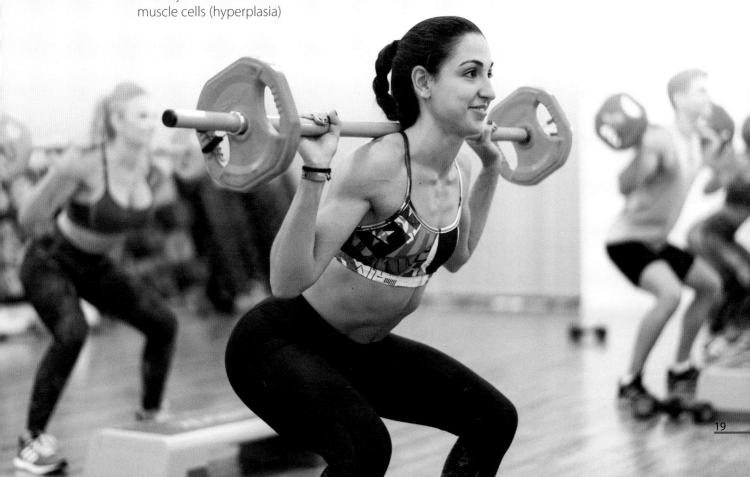

Is Damage Required for Maximizing Adaptation?

Yes, minor damage to muscle fibers appears to be involved in positive adaptations, but a little background information is helpful to keep things in perspective. Although the mantra "no pain, no gain" is bad advice that can result in injury or worse, there is evidence that periodic muscle damage can stimulate muscle to produce more contractile proteins and greater strength. Almost everyone has experienced the acute muscle burning and soreness that accompanies vigorous exercise, especially high-intensity exercise, but those feelings of soreness and discomfort usually subside within minutes after exercise. The muscle soreness that lingers after exercise or arises a day or two later is referred to as *delayed-onset muscle soreness* (DOMS) and indicates damaged muscle.

DOMS is caused by eccentric muscle activity such as downhill running, lowering a heavy weight, or repeated jumps from a platform. DOMS can also occur after any activity that is new and different because virtually all movements involve some eccentric contractions. In each example, ruptured muscle cell membranes and disrupted alignment of contractile proteins occur when muscles resist lengthening, as shown in figure 1.8. Edema (swelling of the damaged area) and inflammation are also hallmarks of DOMS, as fluid and immune cells move from the blood into the muscle to clean up the damage and make way for new proteins.

DOMS temporarily reduces muscle strength because of the damage to contractile proteins and impairs the restoration of muscle glycogen until the damage is repaired. But might periodic DOMS actually be good for stimulating muscle hypertrophy? There are many ways in which muscles become larger and stronger, and it is possible that muscle damage can stimulate these adaptations. Research shows that muscle hypertrophy is greater with eccentric exercise training than with concentric training. Interestingly, muscle hypertrophy has been reported to be greater with rapid-velocity eccentric training, perhaps because of greater

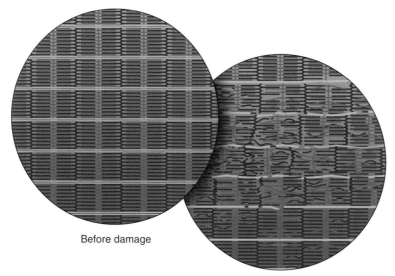

Before damage

Damaged muscle fibers

• Severe damage disrupts the contractile filaments, resulting in an inflammatory response and pain.

• Strength is reduced until the damage is repaired.

▌FIGURE 1.8 Exercise can result in muscle damage that ranges from inconsequential to debilitating.

muscle damage. That finding does not suggest that eccentric training should be the only way to strength train, but this research does underscore the importance of including periodic eccentric training (and DOMS) when increases in mass and strength are desired. However, similar gains in strength and mass have been reported with training programs that do not induce initial muscle damage.

Performance Nutrition Spotlight

Proper nutrition facilitates training adaptations. Water, carbohydrate, protein, fat, vitamins, minerals, and other compounds found in the diet are all important in supporting the many adaptations that occur inside muscle cells.

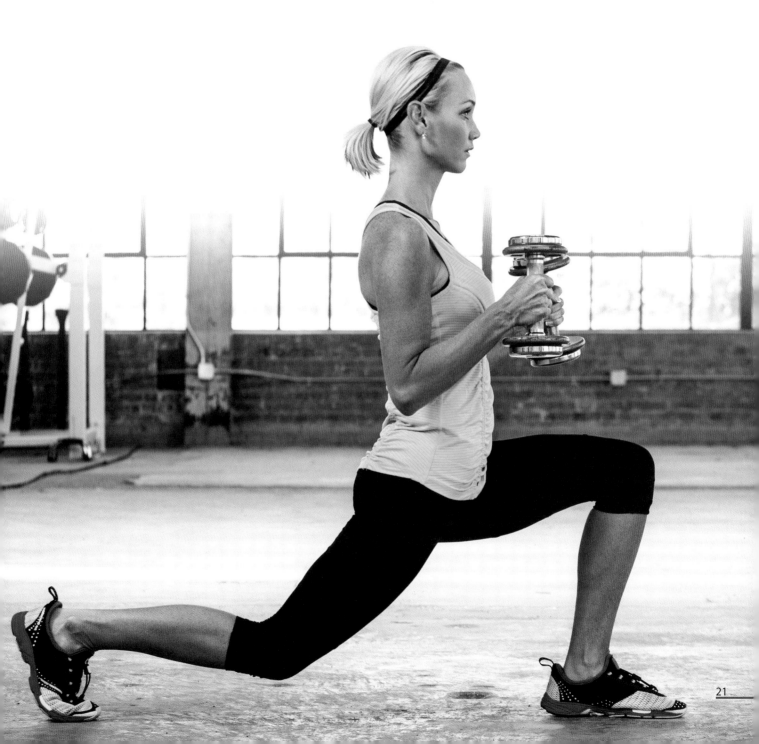

How Do Muscle Cells Get Bigger and Stronger?

All types of exercise result in immediate changes inside and outside muscle cells that serve as signals to promote the production of new functional proteins. In response to aerobic training, the various signals that arise inside muscle cells result in more enzymes involved in aerobic energy production, more mitochondria to enable that energy production, and more myosin filaments with slow-twitch characteristics. In addition to increasing the recruitment of motor units and reducing the normal inhibition of other motor units, strength training signals the nuclei within muscle cells (each skeletal muscle cell contains many nuclei) to produce more contractile proteins and also wakes up some of the usually dormant satellite cells. Muscle cells have been reported to split into two in response to extreme strength training, but cell splitting is not the usual response to training.

At rest and especially during exercise, muscles regularly secrete hundreds of small molecules referred to as *myokines* that travel in the bloodstream and attach to receptors on cell membranes in other tissues and organs. Myokines are thought to influence the function of organs such as bone, cartilage, liver, brain, and fat cells (adipocytes). Myokines are also thought to represent a way in which active muscles can "talk" to distant tissues, alerting them to the needs of muscle cells during exercise, during recovery from exercise, and during the process of adaptation to exercise. *Molecular clocks* inside all cells, including muscle cells, control the secretion of myokines and similar molecules, a function thought to help maintain overall health as well as contribute to healthy aging.

The total number of muscle cells is believed to be fixed at birth.

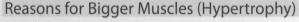

Reasons for Bigger Muscles (Hypertrophy)

- More contractile proteins (actin and myosin)
- More sarcoplasm
- More myofibril units
- More connective tissue
- More intracellular water

What Are Satellite Cells?

All skeletal muscle cells have tiny satellite cells attached to the cell membrane (plasmalemma or sarcolemma). The satellite cells remain inactive until they are activated by strength training, muscle damage, or muscle disease. When needed, the satellite cells spring into action, grow rapidly, and fuse into the neighboring muscle cells, leaving other satellite cells behind to meet future needs (figure 1.9). The proliferation of satellite cells is responsible for most of the muscle growth that occurs early in childhood, during puberty, as a result of training, and in response to muscle damage.

Satellite cells increase the content of contractile proteins in muscle cells and the number of nuclei. Muscle cells are large cells and so require many nuclei to meet the cells' constant need for new proteins. The fitter and stronger you are, the more nuclei you have in your muscle cells. And that may be a good thing as you age because those nuclei appear to stay put over time. These additional nuclei may partly explain why formerly fit people who resume training improve faster than inexperienced exercisers.

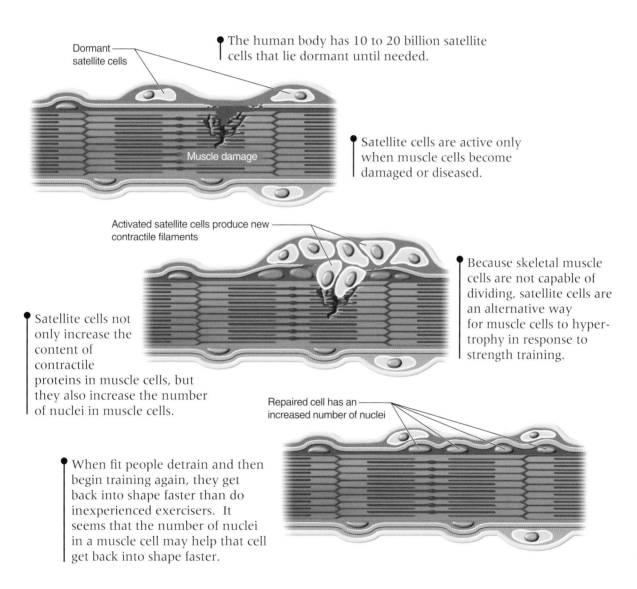

Dormant satellite cells

The human body has 10 to 20 billion satellite cells that lie dormant until needed.

Muscle damage

Satellite cells are active only when muscle cells become damaged or diseased.

Activated satellite cells produce new contractile filaments

Because skeletal muscle cells are not capable of dividing, satellite cells are an alternative way for muscle cells to hypertrophy in response to strength training.

Satellite cells not only increase the content of contractile proteins in muscle cells, but they also increase the number of nuclei in muscle cells.

Repaired cell has an increased number of nuclei

When fit people detrain and then begin training again, they get back into shape faster than do inexperienced exercisers. It seems that the number of nuclei in a muscle cell may help that cell get back into shape faster.

❚ FIGURE 1.9   Satellite cells spring into action to repair damage and promote hypertrophy.

Athletes intuitively understand that consuming protein is important for building strength and mass. The protein needs of most athletes can be easily met by consuming a normal diet, provided that diet has sufficient calories to prevent weight loss and contains a variety of protein foods such as meat, fish, eggs, dairy, nuts, beans, seeds, and whole grains; in other words, a healthy, balanced diet. Even during periods of intense strength training, excess dietary protein is broken down and does not contribute to increases in muscle mass. The American College of Sports Medicine recommends that athletes consume 1.2 to 2.0 grams of protein per kilogram of body weight each day (0.5 to 0.9 grams per pound of body weight each day). In other words, a 150-pound (68 kg) athlete is advised to consume between 75 and 135 grams of protein each day.

What Is the Role of Hormones?

Whenever you are physically active, signals from your brain and from active muscle cells activate the endocrine system to secrete hormones to help support and sustain exercise. The endocrine system includes glands such as the hypothalamus, pituitary, pancreas, thyroid, testes and ovaries, adrenal glands, and even the gastrointestinal tract, all of which secrete hormones that help muscle cells respond to the demands of exercise and adapt to the stress of training.

Steroid and nonsteroid hormones such as testosterone, insulin, insulin-like growth factor (IGF-1), and growth hormone (GH) are among the signals that promote the production of increased functional proteins in muscle cells. Figure 1.10 shows the way that testosterone affects protein production in a muscle cell. Illegitimate use of large doses of testosterone and other anabolic steroids—including prohormones and designer steroids—results in large increases in muscle mass and strength because hormones such as testosterone continuously stimulate the production of contractile proteins.

It is interesting to note that the hormones secreted during and after exercise appear to have little to do with gains in muscle mass and strength. People with more androgen receptors in their muscle cells are most likely to experience muscle hypertrophy with training because more receptors means greater all-day sensitivity to the anabolic hormones that support hypertrophy.

FIGURE 1.10 Steroids and other hormones and growth factors promote the production of a variety of functional proteins inside muscle cells.

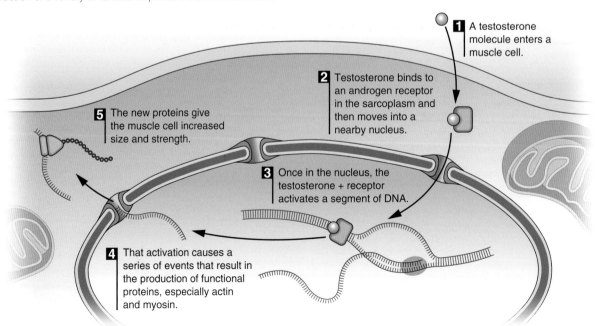

1 A testosterone molecule enters a muscle cell.

2 Testosterone binds to an androgen receptor in the sarcoplasm and then moves into a nearby nucleus.

3 Once in the nucleus, the testosterone + receptor activates a segment of DNA.

4 That activation causes a series of events that result in the production of functional proteins, especially actin and myosin.

5 The new proteins give the muscle cell increased size and strength.

Chapter Summary

- Skeletal muscles contract when motor nerves stimulate groups of muscle cells to contract (motor nerves + muscle cells = motor units).
- Maximal efforts require maximal activation of as many motor units as can be recruited.
- The sliding-filament theory of muscle contraction explains how nerve input results in force production when actin and myosin filaments slide past each other.
- Other proteins in muscle cells—such as titin—also contribute to force production.
- Concentric, eccentric, and isometric contractions all produce force, but in different ways.
- Skeletal muscles are a mix of fast and slow motor units, the proportion of which is determined by genetics.
- Muscles respond to training by adapting to the specific stresses they encounter. For example, strength training increases the amount of contractile proteins within muscle cells, while endurance training increases mitochondrial protein content.
- Genetics establishes the upper limits for strength, speed, power, and endurance.
- Anabolic hormones such as testosterone and growth hormone influence increases in muscle strength and mass in response to training, although increases in those hormones after training or during sleep do not appear to play a major role in that response.

Review Questions

1. Describe how muscles get stronger as a result of proper training.
2. Briefly explain the role of genetics in determining improvements in muscle mass and strength.
3. Define the components of a motor unit.
4. What is the reason for early gains in muscle strength?
5. Describe the primary differences between type I and type II muscle cells.

CHAPTER TWO

Food Really Is Fuel

Objectives

- Discover how food and fluid intake affect performance, recovery, and adaptation.
- Recognize how the nutrients in food provide the energy for muscle contractions and the building blocks for cellular structures.
- Appreciate how muscle cells adjust their energy production to meet the needs imposed by different exercise intensities.

Every muscle contraction is ultimately made possible by the sun. That's because every muscle contraction requires energy, and biological energy on Earth originates with the sun. Energy contained in sunlight is captured by plant life on land and in water and converted through photosynthesis into fuel: carbohydrate, protein, and fat. Animals consume plants (and sometimes each other), capturing the energy contained in plant nutrients for conversion into the carbohydrate, protein, and fat needed for animal growth and daily movement. Humans consume plants and animals to capture the carbohydrate, protein, and fat needed for their growth and daily movement.

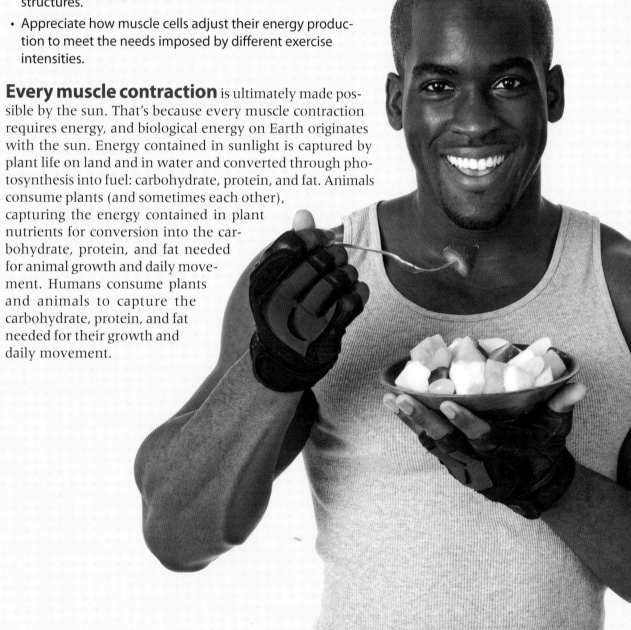

From Food to Energy

The energy contained in carbohydrate, fat, and protein forms the energy required for all metabolic processes, including muscle contraction. From those food sources, your cells create a useable form of energy, a molecule called adenosine triphosphate, or ATP (figure 2.1).

Even though the total amount of ATP in the human body at any given time is only 100 grams (about 3 oz), each day the body produces and uses the equivalent of roughly half of its body weight in ATP. That interesting fact is clear evidence that even when not exercising, the body needs a lot of ATP. How is all that ATP used?

It should be no surprise that ATP production increases dramatically during exercise. The more intense the exercise, the more ATP is needed to sustain muscle contractions. In fact, the body fatigues whenever muscle cells can no longer produce ATP fast enough to fuel muscle contractions. The body also needs ATP for metabolic processes beyond muscle contraction (see sidebar), but during exercise, muscle cells are the main consumers of the ATP.

Why not just eat ATP to maximally fuel muscles for exercise? Unfortunately, that tantalizing proposition doesn't work because, although ATP is a tiny molecule, it's still too large to get across cell mem-

You are what you eat because virtually everything you eat temporarily becomes part of your body.

Each muscle cell contains about one billion ATP molecules, all of which will be used and replaced every 2 minutes.

A molecule of ATP consists of an adenosine group and three inorganic phosphates. The high-energy bonds between the inorganic phosphates store a lot of energy.

When a cell needs energy, the enzyme ATPase breaks one of the phosphates from ATP, releasing energy that can be used by the cell. An ADP molecule — adenosine diphosphate — and an inorganic phosphate molecule are left over.

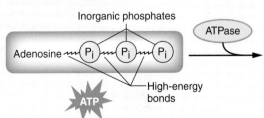
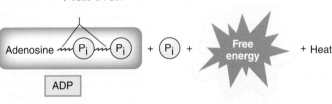

Used for muscle contractions and other metabolic processes.

■ FIGURE 2.1   Adenosine triphosphate (ATP) molecule.

branes. That's actually a good thing because if ATP were able to cross cell membranes, the ATP produced by muscle cells during exercise would leak out of the cells, robbing the cells of the energy needed for muscle contraction. Another problem with ingesting ATP is that most of it would be digested in the stomach and small intestine, so only the bits and pieces of ATP molecules would be absorbed. (By the way, the same limitations exist for eating the enzymes necessary to produce ATP; enzymes are proteins that are digested into their constituent amino acids before being absorbed across the cells of the small intestine into the bloodstream.)

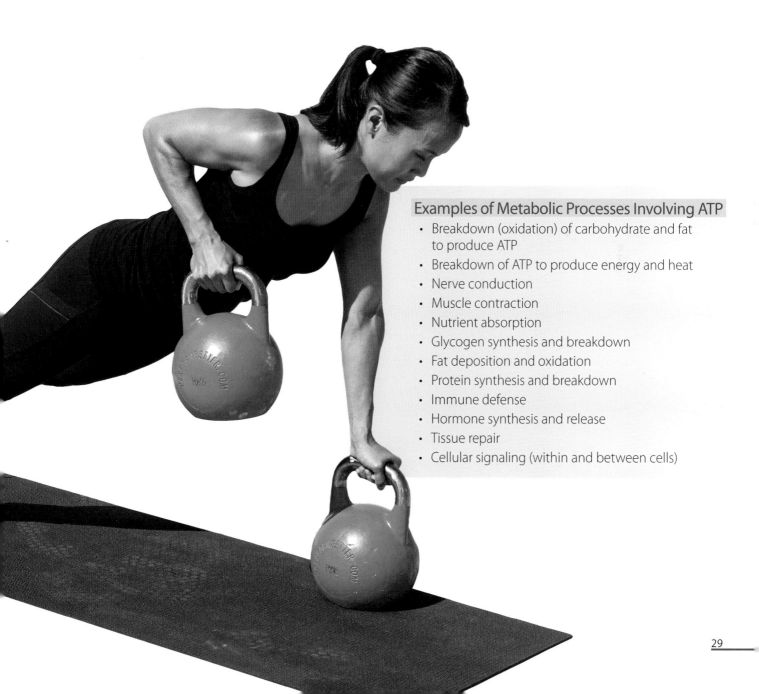

Examples of Metabolic Processes Involving ATP

- Breakdown (oxidation) of carbohydrate and fat to produce ATP
- Breakdown of ATP to produce energy and heat
- Nerve conduction
- Muscle contraction
- Nutrient absorption
- Glycogen synthesis and breakdown
- Fat deposition and oxidation
- Protein synthesis and breakdown
- Immune defense
- Hormone synthesis and release
- Tissue repair
- Cellular signaling (within and between cells)

Although macronutrients (carbohydrate, fat, and protein) can be broken down to form ATP, they are also used by the body in other ways. All the macronutrients consumed on a daily basis meet one of these fates:

- *Carbohydrate* in the form of glucose is broken down (oxidized) inside cells to produce ATP energy, stored as glycogen inside cells to meet future energy needs, circulated in the bloodstream to ensure cells have a steady supply of energy, or used as part of the structure of other molecules (DNA, RNA, glycoproteins, and glycolipids are examples).

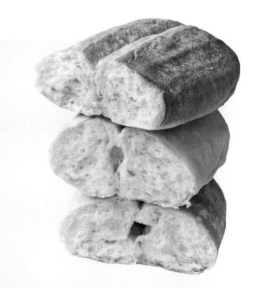

- *Fat* (fatty acids to be precise) can be broken down inside cells to produce ATP energy, stored as triglycerides inside fat cells (adipocytes) as well as other cells, or used in various structural ways, often as the primary component of cell membranes.

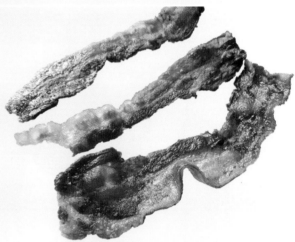

- *Protein* (actually the amino acids that constitute proteins) is primarily used to form various types of proteins throughout the body. But under some circumstances, protein can also be broken down to produce ATP energy or converted into fatty acids or glucose. The body is programmed to minimize the use of protein as energy or for conversion to fatty acids or glucose because protein is a precious commodity. Unlike fat and glucose, excess protein is not stored in the body, so body protein content is protected.

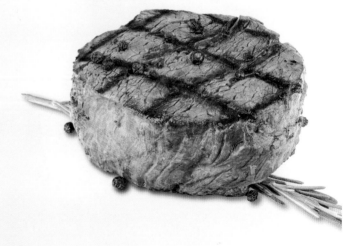

How Do Nutrients Fuel Muscle?

The ATP that muscle cells need for sustaining contractions and performing many other simultaneous functions is produced by three sources, all of which are constantly churning out ATP molecules (figure 2.2).

1. The breakdown of phosphocreatine (PCr)
2. The breakdown of carbohydrate (glucose)
3. The breakdown of fat (fatty acids)

Protein is not a major source of ATP, and that's a very good thing! If protein were used to produce ATP, muscle cells would constantly be breaking down structural and contractile proteins to produce ATP. Fortunately, muscle cells are well designed to break down (oxidize) carbohydrate and fat to produce ATP, sparing the proteins that are so important for other functions inside the cells.

The human body contains 200,000 different kinds of protein.

FIGURE 2.2 Breakdown of carbohydrate, fat, and protein.

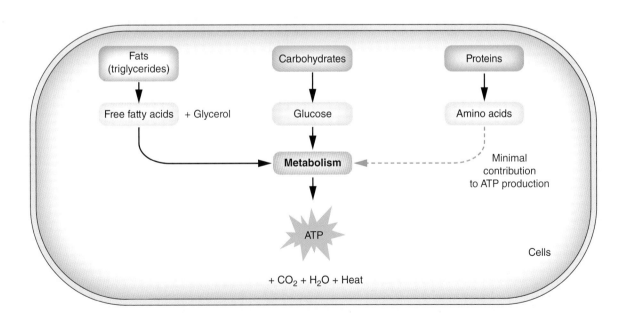

Energy Pathways

As you may know, muscle cells can rely on three ways (three systems or pathways) to produce the ATP needed for muscle contraction. (See figure 2.3.) What is important to remember is that those energy pathways are constantly producing ATP at all times. The intensity of exercise determines which energy pathway produces most of the ATP at any given time.

Muscle cells are metabolically flexible in that they are able to instantly alter the activities of the energy pathways to ensure that ATP supply meets ATP demand.

FIGURE 2.3 In muscle cells, ATP can be produced by the phosphocreatine (PCr) system, anaerobic glycolysis, the citric acid cycle (also known as the Krebs cycle or the tricarboxylic acid [TCA] cycle), and the electron transport chain. All these energy-producing systems work simultaneously and in coordination with one another.

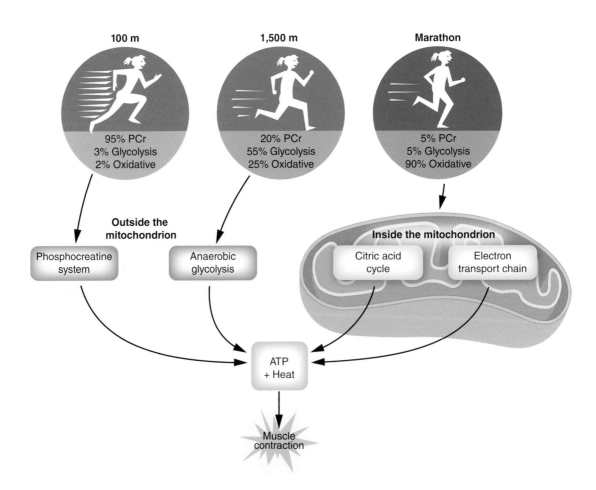

For example, during explosive movements of short duration, such as a 100-meter sprint on the track, most ATP is produced by the *phosphocreatine* (PCr) system, while the breakdown of carbohydrate and fat contributes a comparatively small amount of ATP. The breakdown of phosphocreatine is a simple reaction requiring only one quick step to produce an ATP molecule. Unfortunately, the PCr content of muscle is fairly small, so the PCr system can produce ATP for only short durations (a few seconds) before PCr content falls to low levels.

Anaerobic glycolysis can also produce ATP quickly by breaking down (oxidizing) glucose from the blood and from muscle glycogen stores. (Glycogen is simply a storage form for glucose that enables cells to keep a ready supply of carbohydrate energy close at hand.) The term *anaerobic* is used because this process does not require oxygen. Glycolysis occurs in the sarcoplasm (cytoplasm) of muscle cells that surrounds the contractile filaments so that the ATP produced can be easily used for muscle contraction. Deposits of glycogen are also nearby. Glycolysis is a series of reactions that break glucose molecules in half, capturing the released energy as ATP. The result of breaking glucose in half is two pyruvate molecules (also referred to as pyruvic acid). Pyruvate molecules can quickly be transformed into lactate (lactic acid) molecules during intense exercise or can enter the mitochondria and contribute to the aerobic production of ATP in the citric acid cycle.

Aerobic production of ATP occurs in the many mitochondria in muscle cells. The *citric acid cycle* (also referred to as the Krebs cycle or the tricarboxylic acid cycle) breaks down pyruvate molecules to produce ATP, carbon dioxide (CO_2), and hydrogen ions (H^+). The ATP is shuttled out of the mitochondria and made available for muscle contraction. The CO_2 diffuses out of the muscle cells into the bloodstream, where it is transported to the lungs to be exhaled with each breath, a process detailed in chapter 3. The H^+ ions are used in the *electron transport chain* to produce large quantities of ATP along with water and heat. The electron transport chain is where oxygen (O_2) is used by the muscle cell, and it is also where two H^+ combine with one O to form water, H_2O. The complete oxidation of glucose through glycolysis followed by the citric acid cycle and electron transport chain produces 32 or 33 ATP (depending on whether the original source is muscle glycogen or blood glucose).

Vitamins and minerals play important roles in all metabolic processes leading up to ATP production.

Performance Nutrition Spotlight

Creatine loading can increase the phosphocreatine content of muscle cells and improve performance in the repeated, short-duration explosive movements common in team sport training. The usual approach to creatine loading is to consume 25 grams of creatine each day (or 0.3 g per kg of body weight each day) for one week, followed by 5 grams each day for the duration of the training season.

Muscle cells also use fat to produce ATP. Fat is stored in small quantities inside muscle cells as *intramuscular triglycerides* and in large amounts in fat cells (*adipocytes*). Triglycerides are broken down into three fatty acids and one glycerol molecule, and those fatty acids can be transported in the blood to muscles and other cells to produce ATP. Fatty acids are long chains of carbon molecules along with many hydrogen molecules and a few oxygen molecules. Once the fatty acids are cleaved into two-carbon molecules, those small pieces enter the citric acid cycle following the same path as pyruvate molecules. Because fatty acids are much larger than glucose or pyruvate, each fatty acid produces almost four times as much ATP energy. For example, oxidation of one molecule of a 16-carbon fatty acid called palmitate produces 129 ATP. Unfortunately, fatty acids cannot be broken down very rapidly. As a result, ATP production from fat is important during endurance exercise (and at rest) but far less important during shorter-duration, more intense exercise that requires rapid production of ATP. However, fatty acids are still broken down during intense exercise and do contribute a small amount of ATP to power muscle contractions.

Glucose: The Body's Most Important Fuel

Phosphocreatine stores are limited and fatty acids are oxidized slowly, but carbohydrate (glucose) can be oxidized quickly by anaerobic glycolysis and aerobically in the citric acid cycle to keep up with the demands for ATP during all exercise that lasts longer than 10 seconds. For that reason, carbohydrate is the most important fuel for muscle cells.

Carbohydrate is a catch-all term that refers to a lot of molecules with similar characteristics, from simple sugars such as glucose (blood sugar), fructose (fruit sugar), lactose (milk sugar), and sucrose (table sugar) to more complex forms of carbohydrate such as starches and fibers.

Glucose is the simple sugar—a *monosaccharide*—that the cells rely on every minute of every day to produce ATP. In fact, under normal circumstances the brain and nerves use only glucose as fuel to produce ATP, a reliance that becomes obvious whenever blood sugar level falls too low. Figure 2.4 shows the structure of glucose and some other forms of simple carbohydrate.

Two monosaccharide sugars combined form a *disaccharide;* for example, 1 glucose + 1 fructose = 1 sucrose. When simple sugars are combined in chains longer than two sugars, the resulting molecules are referred to as *oligosaccharides*. A common oligosaccharide used in sports foods and beverages is maltodextrin, short chains of 3 to 10 glucose molecules. Disaccharides and oligosaccharides are quickly digested into their component monosaccharides by digestive enzymes in the mouth and small intestine. The resulting glucose, fructose, and galactose are absorbed through the cells of the small intestine and released

The brain relies solely on glucose for energy. Each day, your brain consumes roughly 130 grams (520 kcal) of glucose.

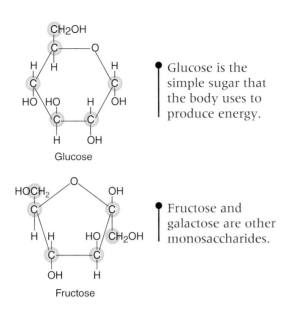

Glucose is the simple sugar that the body uses to produce energy.

Fructose and galactose are other monosaccharides.

Sucrose, the carbohydrate that makes up table sugar (a disaccharide), is formed when fructose and glucose bond together. Similarly, lactose, a sugar found in milk, is formed when glucose and galactose share a bond. Maltose is the combination of two glucose molecules.

FIGURE 2.4   All monosaccharides have the same chemical makeup—$C_6H_{12}O_6$—but slightly different molecular structures.

During intense exercise, muscles can use more than 2 grams of glucose per minute. About half of that can come from glucose ingested during exercise.

into the bloodstream. Very few cells have the enzymes needed for using fructose and galactose, so the liver converts those two sugars into glucose that the liver can store as glycogen or release into the bloodstream to maintain blood sugar levels.

Starches and fibers (and glycogen) are *polysaccharides* composed of thousands of glucose molecules arranged in long branched chains. Starches can be broken down into glucose by a digestive process that starts with enzymes in the mouth and finishes inside the small intestine. These enzymes break large starch molecules into smaller pieces that can be further broken apart by other enzymes into monosaccharides. With fibers such as cellulose, the bonds that hold the glucose molecules together cannot be broken apart; therefore, fibers are not digested and absorbed. Interestingly, many of the bacteria that live in the large intestine (those colonies of bacteria are often referred to as the *microbiome*) can consume fibers to produce the ATP they need to survive. The activity of those bacteria—and the molecules they produce—contribute to overall health.

Keep in mind that regardless of the form of carbohydrate you ingest, glucose is the sugar used by your body. (See figure 2.5.) For instance, if you consume a breakfast of orange juice, cereal, and whole-grain toast, the monosaccharides, disaccharides, oligosaccharides, and polysaccharides in those foods all end up as single glucose molecules in your body.

The speed at which carbohydrate enters the bloodstream and is made available to muscle and other tissues depends in part on how rapidly a meal or snack exits the stomach into the small intestine, where digestion and absorption occur. The more calories you put into the stomach, the slower that food empties into the small intestine.

Whenever you consume sports drinks, carbohydrate gels, and energy bars during exercise, the carbohydrate is quickly absorbed and converted into glucose that muscle cells can extract from the bloodstream and metabolize for ATP. In fact, during intense exercise, muscles can use more than 1 gram per minute from carbohydrate ingested during exercise. That extra energy source helps muscle maintain a high rate of carbohydrate oxidation, improving performance capacity.

What About Fat and Protein?

A performance diet contains a variety of foods and therefore a variety of carbohydrates, fats, and proteins. Figure 2.6 maps out some of the types of fat. Fat is consumed either as individual fatty acids or as triglycerides (three fatty acids connected to one glycerol molecule). Enzymes in the small intestine break apart the triglycerides so that individual fatty acids can be absorbed and distributed in the bloodstream to cells throughout the body (figure 2.7). Cells take up fatty acids for use as part of the cells' membranes, as the building blocks for other molecules, or to break down to form ATP.

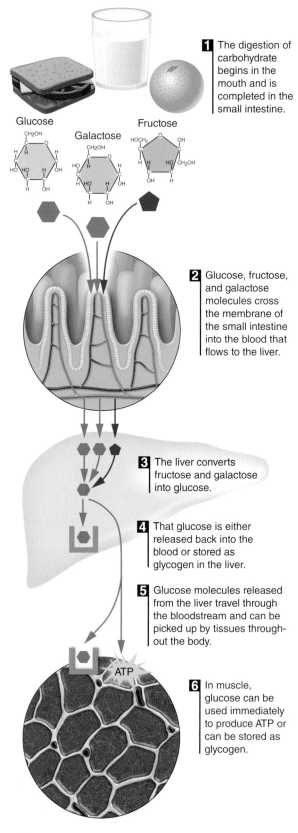

Glucose   Galactose   Fructose

1 The digestion of carbohydrate begins in the mouth and is completed in the small intestine.

2 Glucose, fructose, and galactose molecules cross the membrane of the small intestine into the blood that flows to the liver.

3 The liver converts fructose and galactose into glucose.

4 That glucose is either released back into the blood or stored as glycogen in the liver.

5 Glucose molecules released from the liver travel through the bloodstream and can be picked up by tissues throughout the body.

ATP

6 In muscle, glucose can be used immediately to produce ATP or can be stored as glycogen.

FIGURE 2.5 How carbohydrate is digested, absorbed, and used by the body.

• Fat in food is in the form of triglycerides, which are simply three fatty acids connected to one glycerol molecule. Triglycerides are the form in which fat is stored by plants and animals, including humans.

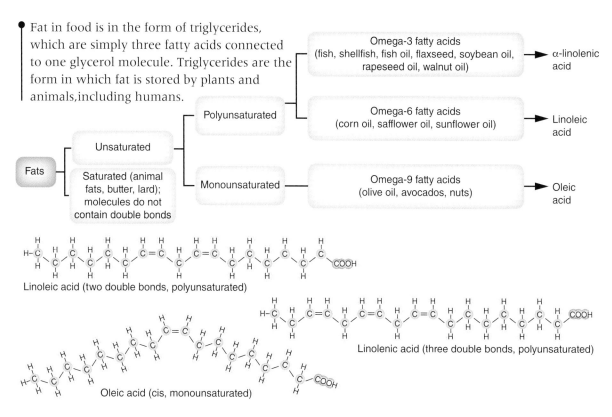

FIGURE 2.6   There are many types of fatty acids that vary in even-numbered lengths from 4 to 28 carbon atoms and in the number of oxygen and hydrogen atoms. Muscles can break down any fatty acid to produce ATP.

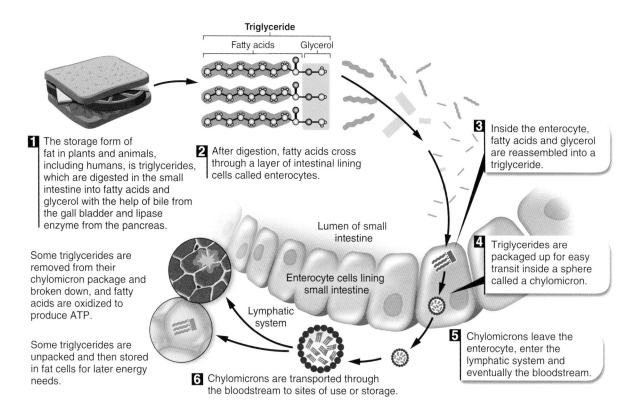

FIGURE 2.7   Fat is broken down in the small intestine and distributed in the blood for use as energy or to be stored.

The protein in foods such as meat, fish, dairy products, vegetables, seeds, and beans is digested with the help of acids and enzymes in the stomach, and enzymes from the small intestine finish the job of breaking protein into individual amino acids. Of the 20 amino acids that the body uses, 9 have to be supplied by food; the other 11 can be synthesized by the body as needed. Those 9 amino acids are referred to as the *essential amino acids*. (See table 2.1.)

When it comes to building and repairing muscle, the essential amino acids are, well, essential. That doesn't mean that essential amino acids are the only amino acids used to build and repair muscle, because all the amino acids are used to create protein. But it does mean that the essential amino acids have to be present for protein building to occur. If you don't eat enough essential amino acids, your body scavenges the needed amino acids by breaking down existing protein, and that is something to avoid.

When it comes to producing ATP inside muscle cells, amino acids are the fuel of *last* choice. After all, why would any cell want to break down its own protein to make ATP? Doing so would degrade the cell's structure and internal functions. That's why cells rely on glucose and fatty acids, not amino acids, to make ATP. Figure 2.8 shows the pathway of protein breakdown in the body.

The daily protein requirement is estimated to be 0.8 gram per kilogram of body weight per day (roughly 0.4 g/lb/day; 60 grams/day for a 150-lb person). At least that's the value for people who aren't very physically active. For athletes and others who exercise more than an hour each day, daily protein needst to rise because more protein is needed for growth and repair of muscle cells. Current recommendations from the American College of Sports Medicine are that athletes should consume 1.2 to 2.0 grams of protein per kilogram of body weight per day (0.5 to 0.9 g/lb/day) to meet the increased needs for muscle growth, repair, and adaptation. Using that math, a 100-pound (45 kg) athlete should consume 50 to 90 grams of protein each day. Even a 300-pound (135 kg) athlete needs only 150 to 270 grams of

TABLE 2.1 **Essential and Nonessential Amino Acids**

Essential	Nonessential
Isoleucine	Alanine
Leucine	Arginine
Lysine	Asparagine
Methionine	Aspartic acid
Phenylalanine	Cysteine
Threonine	Glutamic acid
Tryptophan	Glutamine
Valine	Glycine
Histidine (children)*	Proline
	Serine
	Tyrosine
	Histidine (adult)*

*Histidine is not synthesized in infants and young children, so it is an essential amino acid for children but not for adults.

Reprinted by permission from W.L. Kenney, J.H. Wilmore, and D.L. Costill, *Physiology of Sport and Exercise,* 7th ed. (Champaign, IL: Human Kinetics, 2020), 393.

Each cell in your body contains about 100 million protein molecules. Those molecules represent at least 20,000 different types of proteins.

protein daily. (To keep things in perspective, a 10-ounce (300 g) steak contains about 75 grams of protein.) Ingesting the recommended amount of protein is easy for any athlete who consumes a balanced diet and the same is true for vegetarian and even vegan athletes. In other words, protein powders and amino acid supplements usually aren't needed. However, for athletes who are injured, are on restricted diets (low-calorie or low-carbohydrate diets), or have poor eating habits, a protein supplement or shake can help ensure adequate protein intake at no risk to health.

Research shows that consuming high-protein foods after exercise can boost muscle protein synthesis, giving athletes a jump start on muscle growth and recovery. Equally interesting and of great practical value is that not much protein is needed. It takes only 20 grams of a high-quality protein to maximally boost muscle protein synthesis. In addition, consuming small snacks high in protein every couple of hours throughout the day provides a further boost to muscle protein synthesis. Dairy products appear to be particularly effective at boosting muscle protein synthesis because dairy protein is high in essential amino acids, especially the essential amino acid leucine, which is a metabolic spark for muscle protein synthesis. This is the reason many sport nutrition experts recommend that athletes consume a large glass of chocolate milk after hard workouts (cow's milk contains 1 gram of protein per fluid ounce (30 ml), and the sugar in the chocolate helps to replenish muscle glycogen).

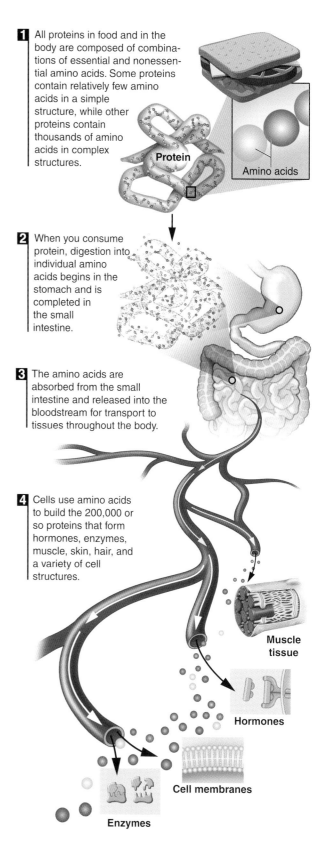

1 All proteins in food and in the body are composed of combinations of essential and nonessential amino acids. Some proteins contain relatively few amino acids in a simple structure, while other proteins contain thousands of amino acids in complex structures.

Protein

Amino acids

2 When you consume protein, digestion into individual amino acids begins in the stomach and is completed in the small intestine.

3 The amino acids are absorbed from the small intestine and released into the bloodstream for transport to tissues throughout the body.

4 Cells use amino acids to build the 200,000 or so proteins that form hormones, enzymes, muscle, skin, hair, and a variety of cell structures.

Muscle tissue

Hormones

Cell membranes

Enzymes

FIGURE 2.8 Damaged or unneeded proteins are broken down into their individual amino acids and can be used for various purposes in the body.

Putting It All Together

Figure 2.9 summarizes the fate of dietary carbohydrate, fat, and protein, and table 2.2 lists the caloric value for each. Carbohydrates, proteins, and fats from food provide the ATP energy needed by all cells and are used to repair, replace, and add new cellular structures, such as the amino acids from food proteins that are used to create new muscle protein.

As noted earlier, all energy pathways continuously produce ATP. The intensity of physical activity determines which energy pathway is the primary producer of ATP. Under normal circumstances, the body stores lots of usable energy in fat, liver, and muscle cells. Figure 2.10 is a pie chart that depicts the various fuel stores in the body.

TABLE 2.2 **The Caloric Value of Macronutrients**

Nutrient	Energy provided
Carbohydrate	4 kcal/gram
Fat	9 kcal/gram
Protein	4 kcal/gram
Alcohol (ethanol)	7 kcal/gram

FIGURE 2.9 Carbohydrates, fats, and proteins in the diet are first digested in the stomach and small intestine before being absorbed into the bloodstream where they either circulate in the blood as an available *"substrate pool"* to be used for metabolism or are stored for later use.

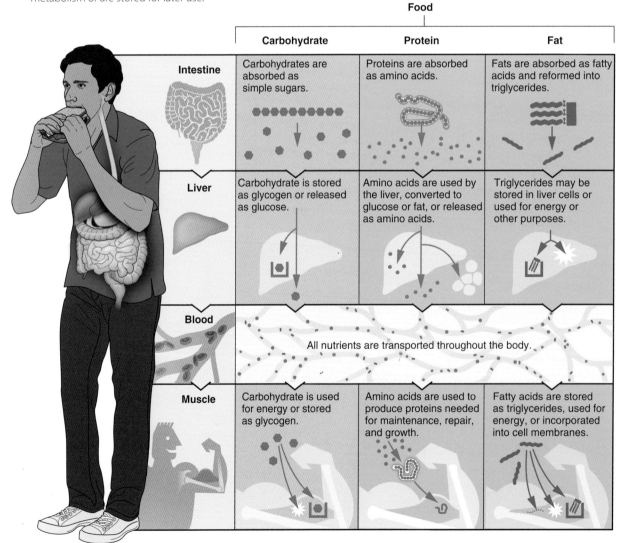

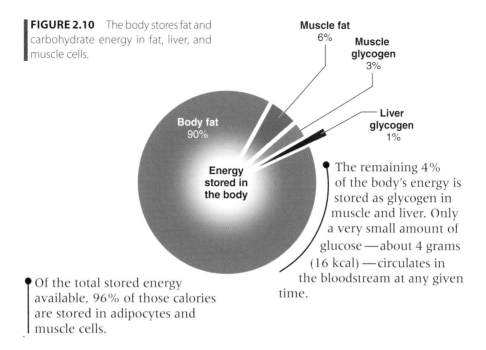

FIGURE 2.10 The body stores fat and carbohydrate energy in fat, liver, and muscle cells.

Of the total stored energy available, 96% of those calories are stored in adipocytes and muscle cells.

The remaining 4% of the body's energy is stored as glycogen in muscle and liver. Only a very small amount of glucose —about 4 grams (16 kcal) —circulates in the bloodstream at any given time.

A quick explanation before getting into the numbers: In scientific literature, 1 Calorie (capitalized) equals 1 kilocalorie (kcal), and technically 1 kilocalorie equals 1,000 calories (lowercased). However, the calorie most people refer to in food is actually 1 kilocalorie. In this book, we'll use Calorie for clarity in scientific contexts and calorie in everyday contexts.

Although you can store more than 2,000 Calories (kcal; see chapter 3 for more information on the energy content of foods and beverages) of energy as muscle glycogen, fat stores amount to more than 75,000 Calories (in a 140-pound [63 kg] person with 12% body fat), so you're well supplied for low-intensity exercise as long as you can consume enough carbohydrate to maintain blood glucose concentration. During prolonged endurance events such as marathons, Ironman triathlons, and ultraendurance competitions, fatty acids can provide a considerable amount of the needed energy (ATP), reducing the demand on blood glucose and muscle glycogen. Maintaining blood glucose by ingesting sports drinks and consuming carbohydrate-rich snacks (e.g., energy bars, carbohydrate gels, pretzels, fruit) ensures that the brain and nerves have a constant supply of glucose from the blood.

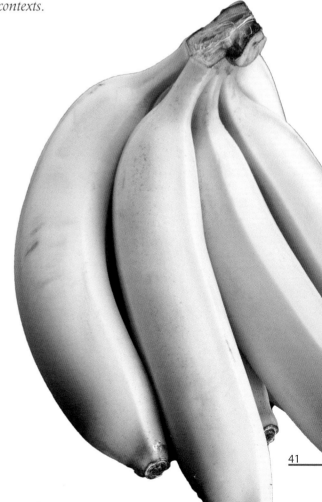

Take a quick look at figure 2.11 and you'll see that the rate at which each energy pathway can produce ATP varies widely, as does the amount of ATP each pathway can produce. The PCr pathway can produce ATP quickly but can't produce much of it. On the other end of the ATP-producing spectrum, fat oxidation produces ATP slowly but can produce it for a long time. The varying capacities for ATP production ensure that cells usually get the ATP they need. One exception is during intense exercise, when the energy pathways can't produce ATP fast enough to fuel muscle contraction, a topic covered in chapter 4. Table 2.3 summarizes the characteristics of the various energy pathways.

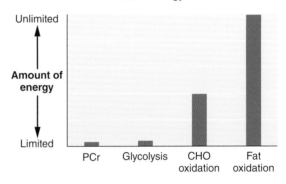

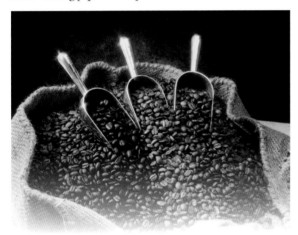

FIGURE 2.11 The rate of energy production and the amount of energy that can be produced vary inversely.

Adapted by permission from W.L. Kenney, J.H. Wilmore, and D.L. Costill, *Physiology of Sport and Exercise,* 7th ed. (Champaign, IL: Human Kinetics, 2020), 69.

Does Caffeine Give You Energy?

Energy drinks and similar supplements are popular products because feeling more energized during the day is appealing and that is especially true when it comes time to train or compete. Most energy drinks and preworkout supplements do contain a source of energy in the form of carbohydrate, but they also contain varying amounts of caffeine (a stimulant to the central nervous system). Although caffeine does not provide metabolic energy in the same way as carbohydrate and fat, ingesting caffeine does increase alertness and mental focus and can improve performance. Energy drinks typically contain 160 to 260 milligrams of caffeine in 16 ounces (475 ml). By comparison, 16 ounces of coffee contains 200 to 300 milligrams of caffeine, and colas have roughly 70 to 120 milligrams of caffeine per 16 ounces. As with everything in the diet, caffeine can be consumed safely in moderation. For athletes and clients who want to use caffeine to improve endurance, strength, or power performance, consuming 100 to 200 milligrams of caffeine 45 to 60 minutes before training or competition should be sufficient.

Regular physical exercise increases muscles' capacity to use fat and carbohydrate to produce ATP because exercise prompts muscles to increase the signaling pathways, enzymes, and mitochondria responsible for ATP production. A proper diet, including adequate hydration before, during, and after exercise, provides the macro- and micronutrients (vitamins and minerals) that all cells require to generate the ATP needed for the function, repair, and growth of cells. Scientists are learning more about the role of many other compounds found in plant (*phytonutrients*) and animal (*zoonutrients*) foods that contribute to overall health, adaptation to training, and performance. Examples include carotenoids, flavonoids, and resveratrol from fruits and vegetables, along with carnitine, coenzyme Q10, and creatine from various meats.

TABLE 2.3 **Characteristics of the Various Energy Supply Pathways**

Energy pathway	Oxygen necessary?	Overall chemical reaction	Relative rate of ATP formed per second	ATP formed per molecule of substrate	Available capacity
ATP-PCr	No	PCr to Cr	10	1	<15 sec
Glycolysis	No	Glucose or glycogen to lactate	5	2-3	~1 min
Oxidative (from carbohydrate)	Yes	Glucose or glycogen to CO_2 and H_2O	2.5	36-39	~90 min
Oxidative (from fat)	Yes	FFA or triglycerides to CO_2 and H_2O	1.5	>100	Days

Courtesy of Dr. Martin Gibala, McMaster University, Hamilton, Ontario, Canada.

Performance Nutrition Spotlight

Consuming 20 to 40 grams of high-quality protein (e.g., dairy, eggs, meat, fish, chicken, and soy) soon after exercise optimizes muscle protein synthesis. Done consistently, this practice leads to greater muscle strength and mass. An interesting side note is that consuming whole milk results in greater muscle protein synthesis than consuming skim milk; likewise, whole eggs are better than egg whites. Scientists are not quite sure why this is so, but the practical implication is that athletes should strive to eat most of their daily calories as whole foods, rather than nutrition supplements.

What About Vitamins and Minerals?

Vitamins are essential nutrients the body cannot make, so there's no doubt that you need to consume vitamins on a daily basis to ensure that all cells are supplied with the substances needed for metabolism—not just energy metabolism but metabolism of all sorts. Even though the body contains roughly 10 thousand trillion cells, each cell needs only a tiny amount of vitamins to operate efficiently. Consuming more vitamins than a cell can use is like having more hammers on a construction site than the workers can use. The extras do no good.

Some vitamins are soluble in water, others in fat. That distinction is important because fat-soluble vitamins (A, D, E, K) are stored and used in liver and fat, whereas water-soluble vitamins (B vitamins, C) are used in the watery environments inside muscle and other cells. All are needed in small amounts to support cell functions. Figure 2.12 is an overview of some of the functions of vitamins and minerals.

Vitamins play an important role in energy metabolism. That's especially true of the B vitamins because they act as cofactors in a variety of enzymatic reactions in the steps that break down glucose and fatty acids to produce ATP.

Some enzymes can perform 1,000 functions per second.

FIGURE 2.12 Some of the functions of vitamins and minerals in the body.

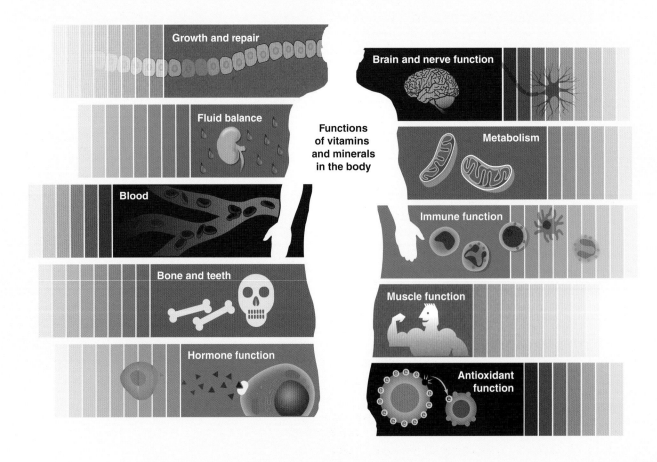

Once each of the muscle cells has enough vitamins to act as cofactors, the body has no choice but to excrete the extra vitamins in the urine. Because enzymes, like all other proteins in the body, break down and are replaced on an ongoing basis, you need to consume small amounts of vitamins every day to ensure that the cells have a steady supply. Table 2.4 lists the recommended daily values for important vitamins and minerals. Consuming the daily values is easily accomplished with a balanced diet. But, as with protein needs, if athletes have poor dietary habits or are on restricted diets, a low-dose multivitamin and mineral supplement can be a low-cost, low-risk way to ensure adequate intake.

As with vitamins, the body needs a small supply of minerals each day because minerals are lost in urine and sweat. Minerals play a variety of roles in the body (figure 2.12). Some minerals are involved in ATP production, while others are involved in nerve conduction, bone formation, red blood cell production, and so on. Although all cells need minerals, the daily need is small and can easily be met by consuming a balanced diet, especially if you're not physically active. Table 2.4 gives general guidelines for mineral intake, but the amount of minerals needed in the diet varies widely because mineral use and loss vary widely, both from day to day and from person to person. Whenever you sweat, mineral loss is increased because sweat contains minerals such as sodium, chloride, potassium, calcium, and magnesium. (Minerals are also referred to as electrolytes or ions because each carries either a positive or negative charge.)

With some athletes, daily sweat loss can be greater than 8 liters, so daily mineral loss will also be high. In most cases, eating enough food energy supplies more than enough minerals to replace sweat mineral losses, so mineral deficiencies are very rare. One possible exception to that statement is the calcium needs of female athletes. Because many females do not consume enough calcium-rich foods to meet the daily recommendation of 1,000 milligrams, and because calcium is lost in sweat, female athletes should be educated on the importance of consuming adequate calcium on a daily basis.

TABLE 2.4 **Daily Values for Vitamins and Minerals**

Vitamin or mineral	Daily values
VITAMINS	
A	5,000 IU
B₁ (thiamin)	1.5 mg
B₂ (riboflavin)	1.7 mg
B₃ (niacin)	Women: 14 mg Men: 16 mg
B₆ (pyridoxine)	2 mg
B₁₂ (cobalamin)	6 mcg
C (ascorbic acid)	60 mg
D (cholecalciferol)	400 IU
E (tocopherols)	30 IU
K (phylloquinone)	80 mcg
Biotin	30 mcg
Folate	400 mcg
Pantothenic acid	10 mg
MINERALS	
Calcium	1,000 mg
Chloride	3,400 mg
Chromium	120 mcg
Copper	2 mg
Iodine	150 mcg
Iron	18 mg
Magnesium	400 mg
Manganese	2 mg
Molybdenum	75 mcg
Phosphorous	1,000 mg
Potassium	3,500 mg
Selenium	70 mcg
Sodium	2,400 mg
Zinc	15 mg

It is now clear that altering the composition and timing of food intake can enhance the adaptations that occur in response to training. For example, purposefully varying the content of muscle glycogen by changing the intensity and duration of training along with the carbohydrate content of the diet and the use (or non-use) of carbohydrate during training can enhance metabolic signals inside muscle cells and thereby improve adaptations to training. (Less clear is whether these strategies consistently improve performance.) These strategies have been shown to stimulate muscle cells to rapidly restore glycogen when adequate carbohydrate is consumed, produce more muscle mitochondria, enhance fat oxidation, and stimulate *angiogenesis* (new capillaries) in muscle. Here are some examples of periodized nutrition strategies:

- *Train high, compete high.* Consume a high-carbohydrate diet with additional carbohydrate intake before, during, and after training to ensure that muscle and liver glycogen content remains high and that muscles—and the gastrointestinal tract—are accustomed to handling carbohydrates consumed during training.
- *Train low, compete high.* Consume a low-carbohydrate diet before, during, and after 7 to 10 days of training and do not emphasize carbohydrate in the diet except for the three days leading up to competition.
- *Recover low, sleep low.* Avoid consuming carbohydrate before, during, and after training and particularly after a hard afternoon or evening workout. Sleeping with low muscle and liver glycogen turns on intracellular signals for glycogen storage when more carbohydrate becomes available.
- *Sleep low, train low.* Complete a hard afternoon or evening training session to lower muscle glycogen stores, restrict carbohydrate intake to ensure that you sleep with low muscle glycogen, then complete a morning training session before consuming carbohydrate to further reduce muscle glycogen. Resume carbohydrate intake after the training session.

Nutrition periodization can parallel training periodization (see chapter 5) to optimize training adaptations. For example, in early season training when many athletes may be trying to shed fat weight, reducing energy intake (calories) and increasing protein intake can help. In midseason training, periodically limiting carbohydrate intake while maintaining energy intake will augment training responses. Leading up to important competitions, a reduced training volume should be combined with a high-carbohydrate diet to maximize energy storage.

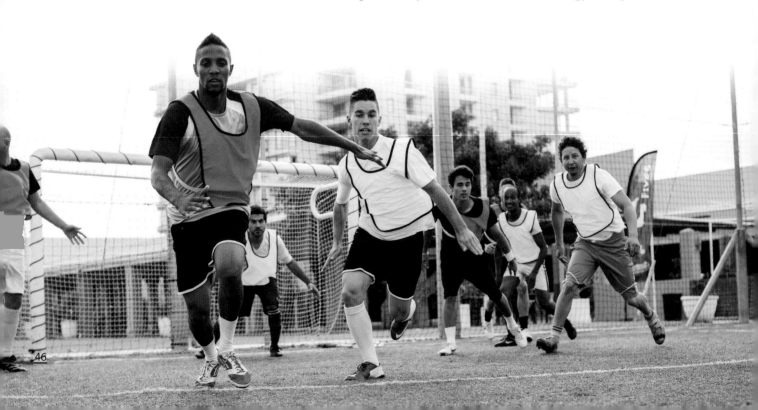

Water Is a Nutrient, Too

For anyone who is physically active, water is arguably the most important nutrient. Water is not only the most biologically active molecule in the body, but it is also the nutrient lost in the greatest amount on a daily basis. Roughly 65% of body weight is plain old water (less as body fat increases), and that figure alone gives a quick indication of how important water molecules must be for bodily functions. (See figure 2.13.)

Even on days when you don't produce a drop of sweat, you still need to drink at least 2 liters of fluid. In fact, the U.S. Institute of Medicine recommends a daily fluid intake of 2.7 liters for females and 3.7 liters for males. These values are estimates of the volumes of fluid American adults should consume each day, but for anyone who breaks a sweat, fluid needs can be much higher. For example, most people are easily capable of losing 500 to 1,000 milliliters (roughly 16-32 oz) of sweat per hour of exercise. A woman who does a hard 2-hour workout and loses 1.5 liters of sweat may have a daily fluid requirement in excess of 4 liters (about 1 gallon). That's a lot of fluid!

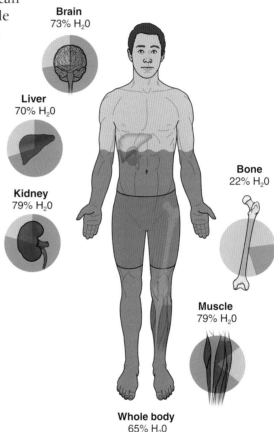

Brain
73% H_2O

Liver
70% H_2O

Kidney
79% H_2O

Bone
22% H_2O

Muscle
79% H_2O

Whole body
65% H_2O

FIGURE 2.13 The human body is about 65% water by weight, but some tissues are composed of even more water.

Drinking for Hydration

Women

2.7 liters per day = 90 ounces per day

20% from food = 18 ounces (0.6 L)

80% from beverages = 72 ounces (2.1 L)

Drink at least 16 ounces (475 ml) with each meal.

Drink at least 8 ounces (237 ml) between meals.

Drink to replace sweat loss.

Men

3.7 liters per day = 125 ounces per day

20% from food = 25 ounces (0.7 L)

80% from beverages = 100 ounces (3.0 L)

Drink at least 24 ounces (700 ml) with each meal.

Drink at least 10 ounces (296 ml) between meals.

Drink to replace sweat loss.

The body's fluid-regulatory mechanisms are pretty good at maintaining proper hydration levels during rest so that at the end of each day, you have much the same volume of water in your body as you had at the start of the day. That's really no small task because, while you are constantly losing fluid, you only periodically drink it. The kidneys continuously produce urine, your skin constantly leaks small quantities of water, and each breath you exhale contains water molecules from the lungs. Those three avenues of fluid loss add up to the recommended 2.7 and 3.7 liters per day. If you eat a diet that contains fruits and vegetables, you can ingest about 20% of daily fluid needs from food. The remaining 80% you have to drink.

The good news is that virtually all beverages count for meeting daily hydration needs (caffeinated beverages, beer, wine, and mixed drinks count, but shots of alcohol do not). With easy access to water, milk, fruit juices, coffee, tea, soft drinks, flavored waters, and sports drinks, you shouldn't have any difficulty staying hydrated. Yet dehydration is still common, especially among those who are physically active. That's because your thirst mechanism is designed to protect you against severe dehydration, not mild dehydration. Fortunately, most fluid intake occurs spontaneously with meals or on other occasions (in meetings or at parties, for example) where drinking occurs in the absence of thirst.

Whenever you become dehydrated by sweating or forgetting to drink enough fluid, two hormones come to the rescue. Dehydration leads to a drop in blood volume and an increase in blood *osmolality* (primarily reflecting the concentration of sodium in the bloodstream). In response, the pituitary gland releases *anti-diuretic hormone* (ADH; also called arginine vasopressin) into the bloodstream and the adrenal

Water Is Constantly Lost From the Body During Rest

- Kidneys are constantly producing urine.
- Water molecules constantly seep through the skin in small quantities.
- Every exhalation is saturated with water molecules.
- Feces accounts for a few ounces of water loss each day.

glands release another hormone called *aldosterone*. ADH promotes thirst and reduces urine production by the kidneys, while aldosterone prompts the kidneys to hold back sodium molecules, further reducing water loss in urine.

Because even a little dehydration impairs a variety of physiological responses as well as physical and even mental performance, it's always better to be well hydrated than dehydrated. For that reason, the best advice is to drink enough fluid (water or sports drinks) during physical activity to minimize loss of body weight. Weight loss during exercise is virtually all sweat loss, so drinking enough to minimize that loss maintains good hydration and provides the fluid needed to maintain blood volume. When you allow yourself to become dehydrated, blood volume shrinks, reducing blood flow to muscles and skin (for heat loss) and causing other negative physiological responses. The simple solution is to drink enough to stay well hydrated (minimize weight loss). That's why it's important to periodically weigh yourself before and after workouts to see if your hydration habits are keeping pace with your sweat losses.

The daily requirement for water also varies widely not only from person to person but also from day to day for the same person. A small, sedentary person living in a cool environment will need less water than a larger, physically active person living in a warm environment. And you need less water on days you don't exercise than on days you do. Your body regulates fluid intake primarily by altering the sensation of thirst and urine production by the kidneys. If you consume too much fluid, thirst diminishes and the kidneys increase urine production. On those occasions when you don't drink enough, thirst is increased and the kidneys reduce urine production.

Most of the fluid consumed on a daily basis comes from beverages, and a smaller amount (about 20%) comes from food. The U.S. Institute of Medicine estimates that adult men should consume 125 ounces (3.7 L) of water each day (100 oz from beverages, 25 oz from foods). For adult women, the value drops to 90 ounces per day (2.7 L; 72 oz from beverages; 18 oz from foods). Those values

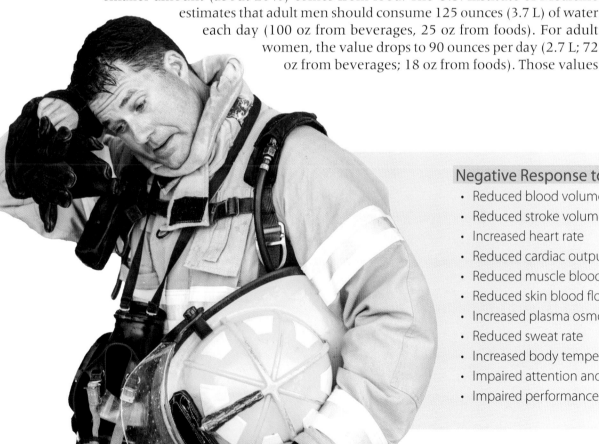

Negative Response to Dehydration

- Reduced blood volume
- Reduced stroke volume
- Increased heart rate
- Reduced cardiac output
- Reduced muscle blood flow
- Reduced skin blood flow
- Increased plasma osmolality
- Reduced sweat rate
- Increased body temperature
- Impaired attention and focus
- Impaired performance

are only estimates of the daily requirements for most adults. Athletes, workers, soldiers—all who work up a sweat—have an increased daily requirement of water that will likely exceed those values. In fact, some people may need to drink 2 gallons or more each day (7.5 L) simply because they sweat a lot.

When sweat losses are extremely high, as can be the case during ultramarathons, Ironman-distance triathlons, and two-a-day practices, a lot of sodium is lost from the body. Under those circumstances, drinking large volumes of plain water will cause the sodium level of the blood to drop below normal, a condition known as *hyponatremia*. The same thing can happen if a resting person drinks a large volume of water quickly. Because you can drink faster than your kidneys can produce urine, the blood sodium level is temporarily diluted. Usually this is not a problem and blood sodium gradually returns to normal as the excess water is excreted by the kidneys. But when the drop in blood sodium is large, swelling of the brain occurs, a condition that can lead to seizures, coma, and death. Exercise-associated hyponatremia is not common, but all sport health professionals should be aware of the possibility and educate physically active people to drink enough fluid to minimize weight loss but avoid extreme overdrinking.

Performance Nutrition Spotlight

Some athletes experience annoying gastrointestinal symptoms such as bloating, burping, and gurgling, not only during exercise but also throughout the day. If such symptoms persist, the best first step is to consult a physician. Also, athletes can try to restrict certain foods to see if the symptoms subside. Some people have found success by reducing or eliminating wheat products (to restrict gluten intake). Others have found relief by restricting the consumption of foods with fermentable (poorly absorbed) carbohydrate, referred to as *FODMAPs*, short for fermentable oligosaccharides, di- and monosaccharides, and polyols (sugar alcohols such as sorbitol, mannitol, and xylitol). Common FODMAP foods are asparagus, cauliflower, broccoli, black beans, kidney beans, onions, peas, and mushrooms.

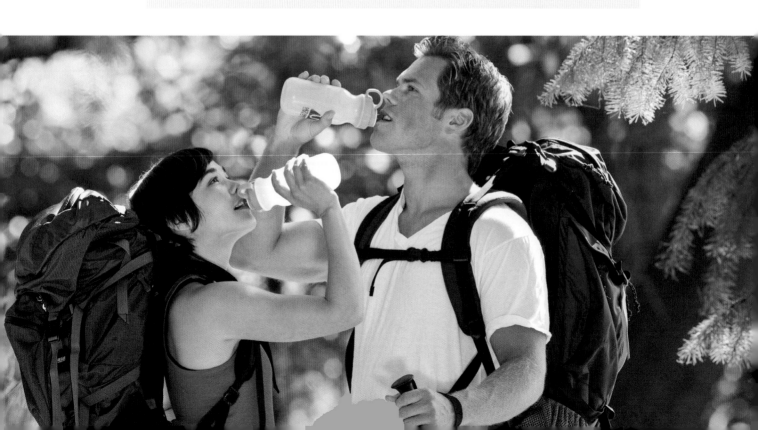

Chapter Summary

- The nutrients and energy (calories) contained in food are essential to growth and development, the capacity for physical activity, and the ability to adapt to that activity.
- Carbohydrates, proteins, and fats are macronutrients that provide energy to active muscles and all other cells and are needed by cells to perform many other functions vital to life.
- Vitamins and minerals are micronutrients needed in small amounts to support a variety of cell functions.
- The role of phytonutrients and zoonutrients from plant and animal foods are not fully understood but appear to be important in overall nutrition.
- The metabolism of carbohydrate and fat supplies the ATP required for muscle contraction and other cell functions.
- Food proteins provide the amino acids needed to repair and rebuild muscle and other structures throughout the body.
- Anaerobic and aerobic energy-producing pathways supply muscle cells with ATP.
- Glucose from carbohydrates in the diet is the most important fuel for muscles and the brain.
- A varied, balanced diet can provide all the nutrients athletes need to perform, recover, and adapt.
- Preventing dehydration is critical to protecting performance.

Review Questions

1. Describe one difference between the use of carbohydrate and the use of fat in the production of ATP molecules during exercise.
2. Explain why we cannot simply eat a dietary supplement containing ATP to gain more energy.
3. Identify one reason glucose is the body's most important fuel.
4. List three examples of molecules that are carbohydrates.
5. Explain why essential amino acids are called essential.

CHAPTER THREE

Muscles Need Oxygen

Objectives

- Understand how the heart, lungs, blood, and vasculature deliver oxygen to cells.
- Learn how oxygen from the air you breathe allows for the aerobic production of ATP.
- Appreciate how regular physical activity increases the capacity of the cardiovascular system to support improved performance.

Oxygen is the third-most abundant element in the universe (hydrogen and helium are first and second). In fact, oxygen makes up most of your body mass because the human body is mostly water—H_2O—and because oxygen molecules are also part of protein, fat, carbohydrate, and many other molecules in the body.

Cells rely on oxygen for the unending production of ATP molecules, which are essential for cell functions, including muscle contractions. Oxygen in the air is continuously replenished by oxygen released from plants as a by-product of photosynthesis, the process plants use to produce ATP.

The air you breathe is 21% oxygen (O_2) (20.93%, to be precise). Most of the air is nitrogen (N_2; 78%) with a pinch of argon (0.9%), and carbon dioxide (CO_2; 0.04%). At sea level, the atmospheric pressure ensures that lungs are exposed to enough O_2 molecules with each inhalation that breathing feels easy, especially at rest. At altitude, such as when climbing Mt. Everest, the lower partial pressure of oxygen in the air impairs endurance performance because altitude limits the amount of oxygen that can be delivered to muscles. On Mt. Everest, where the atmospheric pressure is only 33% of that at sea level, the O_2 molecules are spread so far apart that it's difficult to catch a breath, even at rest. The air at the peak of Mt. Everest still contains 21% oxygen, but the atmospheric pressure is low because at 29,028 feet (8,848 m), there is much less air above to create pressure. As a result, breathing has to be very rapid to introduce enough oxygen into the lungs to satisfy even the low metabolic needs at rest. This simple fact is why most mountaineers rely on supplemental oxygen at very high altitudes.

How Does Oxygen Get to Muscles?

The human body is obviously well equipped to extract oxygen from inhaled air and deliver that oxygen to all cells in the body, including very active muscle cells. That process is actually very simple in concept, even though it's quite complicated in detail.

The lungs allow oxygen from inhaled air to pass across the very thin membranes in the depths of the lungs and enter the bloodstream. At the same time, carbon dioxide that was produced by muscle and other cells leaves the blood by passing across the same lung membranes and being exhaled from the body. This exchange is illustrated in figure 3.1.

Only some of the oxygen in inhaled air passes across the lungs into the blood. At the same time, carbon dioxide is released from the blood and enters the lungs to be exhaled. The movement of those two gases—O_2 and CO_2—depends on their concentrations and their diffusion coefficients. The *diffusion coefficient* is a measure of how quickly a substance tends to move across a membrane such as the lining of the lung alveoli. For example, even though CO_2 is in low concentration in the blood flowing through the lungs, it moves easily from the blood into the lungs because CO_2 has a high diffusion coefficient: 20 times greater than O_2.

> Oxygen is so critical to survival that all nucleated cells in the body have the ability to sense oxygen.

FIGURE 3.1   The exchange of oxygen and carbon dioxide at the lungs. Oxygen binds to hemoglobin in the blood. Iron is an important part of each hemoglobin molecule.

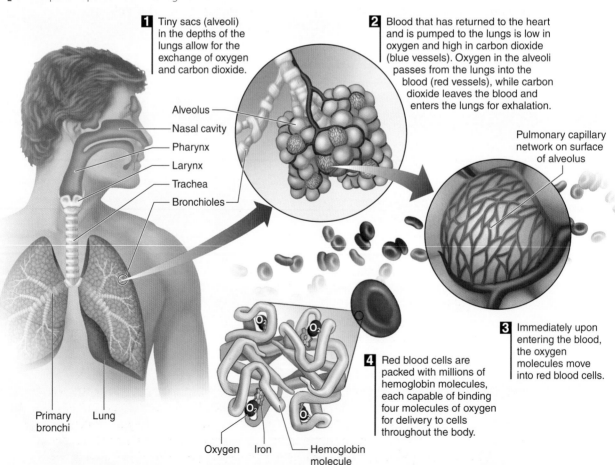

1 Tiny sacs (alveoli) in the depths of the lungs allow for the exchange of oxygen and carbon dioxide.

2 Blood that has returned to the heart and is pumped to the lungs is low in oxygen and high in carbon dioxide (blue vessels). Oxygen in the alveoli passes from the lungs into the blood (red vessels), while carbon dioxide leaves the blood and enters the lungs for exhalation.

Alveolus
Nasal cavity
Pharynx
Larynx
Trachea
Bronchioles

Pulmonary capillary network on surface of alveolus

3 Immediately upon entering the blood, the oxygen molecules move into red blood cells.

4 Red blood cells are packed with millions of hemoglobin molecules, each capable of binding four molecules of oxygen for delivery to cells throughout the body.

Primary bronchi   Lung

Oxygen   Iron   Hemoglobin molecule

When oxygenated blood reaches muscle cells, the bond between oxygen and hemoglobin molecules loosens for a variety of reasons that need not be described here. When the red blood cells pass single file through the tiny capillaries that surround muscle cells (figure 3.2), oxygen molecules are released from hemoglobin and diffuse into the muscle cells. The carbon dioxide produced by the muscle cells diffuses into the bloodstream for transport not as CO_2 but as bicarbonate ion (HCO_3^-) that is converted back into CO_2 gas in the lungs, where it is exhaled. A small amount of oxygen is dissolved in the blood plasma, but that amount is only a tiny fraction of the oxygen that is transported by hemoglobin.

Once inside muscle cells, the oxygen can either bind to *myoglobin* (a protein similar to hemoglobin that enables muscle cells to store a small amount of oxygen) or enter the mitochondria to be used in the electron transport chain to accept the H^+ ions produced by the oxidation of carbohydrate and fat. Before binding with oxygen to form H_2O, the H^+ ions are used in the mitochondria's electron transport chain to produce ATP. The complete oxidation of carbohydrate and fat produces the same products: ATP, H_2O, CO_2, and heat.

The process by which carbohydrate and fat are oxidized to produce ATP is referred to as *internal respiration* because it occurs inside cells. The delivery of oxygen from the lungs to the cells is called *external respiration*.

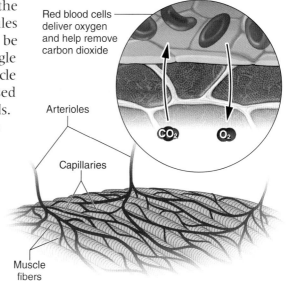

Red blood cells deliver oxygen and help remove carbon dioxide

Arterioles

Capillaries

CO_2 O_2

Muscle fibers

FIGURE 3.2 Muscle cells are supplied by tiny capillaries that deliver oxygen and nutrients and remove waste products such as carbon dioxide and lactic acid.

The Role of Iron in Oxygen Transport

Even though the human body contains only 3 to 4 grams of iron, that small amount plays a variety of essential roles. The iron in each hemoglobin molecule binds oxygen for transport; in fact, the red color of blood is due in part to those iron molecules. Myoglobin in muscle cells also contains iron molecules; myoglobin serves as a way station for oxygen molecules on their short journey from the red blood cells into the mitochondria. In addition, iron molecules are important for the function of many enzymes.

Iron is a mineral needed in small amounts on a daily basis (18 mg per day). Red meat, beans, fish, and leafy vegetables are good sources of iron. Some female athletes are prone to iron deficiency because of iron loss during menstruation combined with low iron intake in their diets. If iron deficiency becomes severe, true anemia (an abnormally low hemoglobin level) can result. Iron deficiency and anemia are far more common in females than in males.

Measuring the iron content in blood is not useful in determining a person's iron status, but other measures such as *plasma ferritin* (the storage form of iron) are used to determine whether someone is iron deficient. If iron stores become too low, the bone marrow has a difficult time maintaining normal hemoglobin production for red blood cells, and iron-deficiency anemia can result. It is possible for athletes to have iron deficiency without anemia; some estimates indicate that 20% to 25% of female athletes are iron deficient (below-normal plasma ferritin levels). Whether or not performance is adversely affected by iron deficiency is a matter of debate, but there is no doubt that iron deficiency is abnormal and should be addressed through changes in diet and perhaps daily consumption of an iron supplement.

Reference: Rowland, T. (2012). Iron deficiency in athletes. *American Journal of Lifestyle Medicine, 6*(4):319-327.

As you become more aerobically fit, your cardiorespiratory system's capacity to deliver oxygenated blood to active skeletal muscle cells improves (see table 3.1). Evidence of that improvement is seen as an increased maximal oxygen consumption ($\dot{V}O_{2max}$), which is measured by a laboratory test that requires participants to exercise at increasing workloads to exhaustion (more about this later). Lung function changes with training, as does heart function. In the heart, the most important change is an increase in *cardiac output,* which means the heart is capable of pumping more blood each minute. Improved fitness also causes blood volume to increase, supporting the increase in cardiac output. In addition, muscle cells increase their capacity to use oxygen. All these changes and more enable the increase in $\dot{V}O_{2max}$ and improved aerobic performance. Figure 3.3 is an overview of how the lungs, heart, blood, and vasculature work together to deliver oxygen and remove carbon dioxide from all cells.

The body actually has two pumps that move blood to and from the heart. The heart itself is the most obvious pump, but the contraction of skeletal muscles is the second pump that ensures that blood is pushed back to the heart.

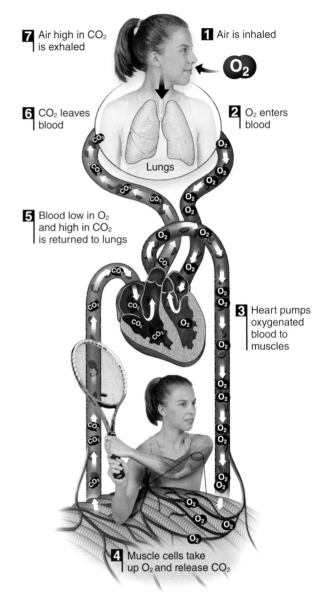

7 Air high in CO_2 is exhaled

1 Air is inhaled

O_2

6 CO_2 leaves blood

2 O_2 enters blood

Lungs

5 Blood low in O_2 and high in CO_2 is returned to lungs

3 Heart pumps oxygenated blood to muscles

4 Muscle cells take up O_2 and release CO_2

FIGURE 3.3 All types of exercise rely on the aerobic production of ATP. The heart, lungs, blood, and vasculature work together to deliver oxygen and remove carbon dioxide.

TABLE 3.1 **Cardiorespiratory Adaptations to Training**

The heart and lungs (cardiorespiratory system) adapt to training as a result of these changes:	Muscle blood flow improves due in large part to these changes:
Increased maximal and submaximal pulmonary ventilation (the volume of air moving through the lungs)	Larger blood volume
Increased blood flow from the heart to the lungs	More arterioles (arteriogenesis)
Increased blood flow to the upper regions of the lungs	More capillaries (capillary angiogenesis)
Increased size and volume of the left ventricle	Recruitment of dormant capillaries
Increased stroke volume	More efficient distribution of blood flow to active muscle cells
Increased cardiac output	Better redistribution of blood from less active tissue to active muscle cells

How Does Oxygen Use Relate to Metabolic Rate?

The body's capacity to use oxygen is a measure of health and fitness. Elite endurance athletes have a large capacity to use oxygen, and that is reflected in their very high maximal oxygen consumption values. At the other end of the spectrum are those with poor physical fitness and very low $\dot{V}O_{2max}$ values.

Measurements of oxygen consumption are used to determine how much oxygen a person is using each minute at rest and during various types, intensities, and durations of exercise. Not only is *maximal* oxygen consumption an indication of aerobic fitness, oxygen consumption measured during an activity allows scientists to calculate the *energy cost* (caloric cost) of that activity (which is why oxygen consumption testing is also referred to as *indirect calorimetry*). Energy cost (also known as *energy expenditure*) is expressed in *kilocalories* (kcal; also called Calories). For example, for a 154-pound (70 kg) person, the energy cost of running at 7.5 miles per hour is roughly 14 kilocalories (kcal or Calories) per minute, a value determined by oxygen consumption testing. The caloric values assigned to different activities such as housework, walking, tennis, and cycling are determined by measuring oxygen consumption.

Metabolic Rate at Rest and During Exercise

You might have heard someone say, "She's thin so she must have a high metabolic rate." *Metabolic rate* is simply the rate at which the body uses energy. In other words, metabolic rate, energy expenditure, and oxygen consumption can be considered synonyms. You'll also hear other terms such as *resting metabolic rate* (RMR) and *basal metabolic rate* (BMR) used to refer to the energy expenditure at rest. RMR and BMR are measured in slightly different ways, but the values are similar. In both cases, measures of oxygen consumption can be used to estimate resting metabolic rate.

As an example, consider the RMR for a 128-pound (58 kg) woman with 24% body fat. A person of this size and body composition will consume about 250 milliliters (0.25 L) of oxygen every minute at rest. There are 1,440 minutes in a day, so her oxygen consumption would be 0.25 liter per minute $\times$ 1,440 minutes per day, or 360 liters of oxygen per day. How do 360 liters of oxygen convert to calories? For that conversion, you need to know that each liter of oxygen is equivalent to 4.8 Calories (under these circumstances). At this point, the math is simple: This woman's RMR is estimated to be 360 liters per day × 4.8 Calories per liter, or 1,728 Calories (kcal) per day. Now you know the number of calories this woman must consume to maintain her current body weight. If she is physically active, the energy cost of her daily activity is added to her RMR to estimate her total energy (caloric) needs.

Oxygen consumption—abbreviated as $\dot{V}O_2$—increases whenever the body needs more oxygen to meet its metabolic needs. It should be no surprise that oxygen consumption at rest is low compared to oxygen consumption during any type of physical activity. Oxygen consumption at rest depends mostly on a person's body size (specifically, on fat-free mass and body surface area). In other words, resting oxygen consumption is higher in larger people than in smaller people because larger people have more cells, all of which require oxygen to function. Once we become active, the more intense the activity, the higher the oxygen consumption. Not surprisingly, the higher your heart rate, the greater your oxygen consumption.

You might have heard the term *MET* (for *metabolic equivalent of training*) used to refer to levels of exercise intensity. One MET is roughly the equivalent to the energy (oxygen) cost of sitting quietly, which is 1 kcal per kilogram of body weight per hour (1 kcal/kg/hr; about 3.5 ml O_2/kg/min). So, an activity that requires 5 METs requires 5 times the energy of sitting quietly. (See the sidebar Factors That Affect Resting Metabolic Rate to learn how RMR can vary from the 1 kcal/kg/hr value used to establish 1 MET.)

Performance Nutrition Spotlight

One of the most important adaptations to training is the increase in blood volume that aids oxygen delivery to active muscles. Becoming dehydrated drastically reduces blood volume, effectively negating that important benefit to training.

$\dot{V}O_{2max}$ and What It Means

Maximal oxygen consumption ($\dot{V}O_{2max}$) is a measure of the body's maximal capacity to use oxygen. It is measured as milliliters of oxygen used per kilogram of body weight per minute, which may range from less than 20 ml/kg/min in very deconditioned people to over 90 ml/kg/min in some elite male endurance athletes. During a maximal exercise test, $\dot{V}O_{2max}$ occurs when the amount of oxygen the person is using does not increase any further in response to increasing exercise intensity. As you become more aerobically fit, muscles increase their capacity to use oxygen. That change allows you to exercise at higher intensities without fatiguing. See figure 3.4 for an example of how one person had a 30% increase in $\dot{V}O_{2max}$, from 44 to 57 ml/kg/min, as a result of training. This magnitude of increase in $\dot{V}O_{2max}$ is fairly typical and generally occurs after 12 to 18 months of proper training.

After a year or so of training, $\dot{V}O_{2max}$ reaches a plateau and does not increase further. But endurance performance can continue to improve because with training it's possible to exercise at a greater percentage of $\dot{V}O_{2max}$. Imag-

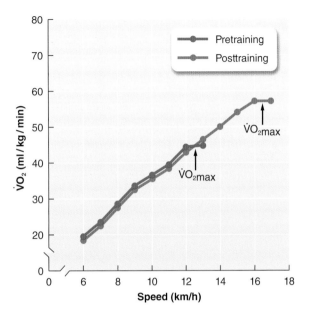

FIGURE 3.4 Maximal oxygen consumption increases with proper training. After 12 to 18 months of training, there are no further increases in $\dot{V}O_{2max}$ in most people.

Reprinted by permission from W.L. Kenney, J.H. Wilmore, and D.L. Costill, *Physiology of Sport and Exercise*, 7th ed. (Champaign, IL: Human Kinetics, 2020), 269.

Factors That Affect Resting Metabolic Rate

The largest part of daily energy (caloric) needs is represented by the energy required to fuel resting metabolism. In other words, if all you did was lie in bed all day, all the cells in your body would still break down glucose and fatty acids to produce the ATP required to meet the resting energy needs of each cell. Larger bodies typically need more energy than smaller bodies, so resting metabolic rate (RMR) is understandably greater for larger people than for smaller people.

According to several studies, the RMR for adult men is calculated to be 0.892 kcal/kg/hr; for females, the value is 0.839 kcal/kg/hr. Keep in mind that these values are just good estimates based on a lot of research and take only body weight into consideration. As it turns out, the same research shows that RMR decreases with age as muscle mass decreases, fat mass increases, and the metabolic rate of organs such as the liver and kidneys gradually declines. RMR is also lower in overweight and obese people than it is in normal-weight people. For example, normal-weight women had an RMR of 0.926 kcal/kg/hr compared to 0.721 kcal/kg/hr in obese women. The values were 0.960 and 0.791 in normal-weight and obese men, respectively. Fat is a low-metabolic-rate tissue, while muscle has a comparatively higher resting metabolic rate. For that reason alone, adding muscle and losing fat increase RMR.

The moral of this story is that maintaining a high RMR as you age depends largely on maintaining muscle mass and keeping body fat at normal levels. Happily, both of those goals are attainable through regular physical activity.

Reference: McMurray, R.G., et al. (2014). Examining variations of resting metabolic rate of adults. *Medicine and Science in Sports and Exercise*, 46(7):1352-1358.

ine that a runner is able to run for an hour at 80% of her $\dot{V}O_{2max}$. With proper training, she might then be able to run for an hour at 86% of her $\dot{V}O_{2max}$, enabling her to run at a faster speed even though her $\dot{V}O_{2max}$ has not increased.

Many elite endurance athletes have very high $\dot{V}O_{2max}$ values: for women, >70 ml/kg/min; for men, >85 ml/kg/min.

There's no doubt that highly fit people have above-average $\dot{V}O_{2max}$ values. But $\dot{V}O_{2max}$ alone is not a good predictor of endurance performance. Also important to performance is the percentage of $\dot{V}O_{2max}$ that can be sustained over time, as in the previous example. That level of effort is often referred to as the *lactate threshold*. The lactate threshold simply refers to the highest exercise intensity that can be sustained without an accumulation of lactic acid in the bloodstream. Even without the laboratory procedures required for measuring $\dot{V}O_{2max}$ and lactate threshold, experienced athletes know how hard they can push themselves and will lower the intensity before exercise becomes unsustainable.

In addition to the lactate threshold, other terms used to describe the highest level of sustainable exercise include *anaerobic threshold, ventilatory threshold, gas-exchange threshold, functional threshold power,* and *critical power*. The definitions of these measures vary, but all refer to tests used to distinguish moderate, heavy, and severe exercise intensities.

Measuring maximal oxygen consumption requires special equipment and experienced staff, so most athletes have to depend on improvements in training and competition as evidence that their aerobic capacity or lactate threshold has improved. After all, the result of improved performance is far more important than knowing how much an athlete's maximal oxygen consumption might have risen with training. A variety of aerobic fitness tests have been developed to estimate maximal oxygen consumption. For example, 1.0- or 1.5-mile run times on a track as well as treadmill and cycle ergometer tests can be used to estimate maximal oxygen consumption and assess changes in aerobic fitness.

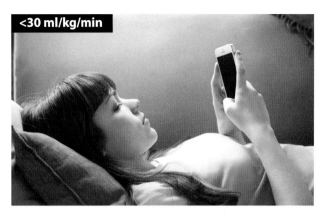
<30 ml/kg/min

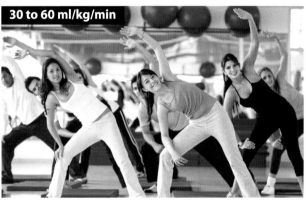
30 to 60 ml/kg/min

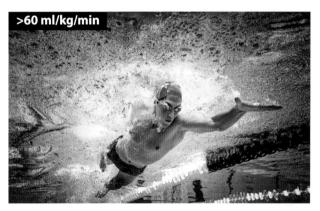
>60 ml/kg/min

Performance Nutrition Spotlight

Oxygen delivery to muscles depends in large part on having normal hemoglobin levels. Because oxygen molecules attach to iron molecules in hemoglobin, consuming enough iron in the diet is important to replace daily iron losses, especially for female athletes. The foods you eat contain iron in two forms: heme iron and non-heme iron. Animal meat contains a combination of the two forms, while dairy, eggs, and vegetables contain non-heme iron. Heme iron is absorbed more efficiently than non-heme iron. Female athletes, vegan or vegetarian athletes, and athletes spending an extended time at altitude should be sure to consume a varied diet to ensure ample iron intake. They should also consider taking a daily iron supplement, as well as vitamins C and B_{12} to aid iron absorption.

Other Terms You Should Know

Before turning your attention to how training affects the body's ability to use oxygen, become familiar with four terms associated with oxygen consumption. The first term is *respiratory exchange ratio* (RER). Although RER has little practical value outside the laboratory, you should be aware of what it means and how it is used. Without getting too technical, RER is the ratio between oxygen use and carbon dioxide production, calculated by dividing the volume of CO_2 produced each minute by the volume of O_2 used each minute:

$$RER = \frac{\dot{V}CO_2}{\dot{V}O_2}$$

RER is used to estimate how much fat and carbohydrate are oxidized to produce ATP. Your body is always using both carbohydrate and fat to produce ATP, but the ratio of the two fuel sources changes depending on exercise intensity. At

Why Does Maximal Heart Rate Decline With Age?

One of the physiological changes that occur with aging is a decline in maximal heart rate. In fact, maximal heart rate declines roughly 1 beat per minute per year. That simple fact is the basis for the most common equation for estimating maximal heart rate: $HR_{max} = 220 - age$. However, that equation provides only a rough estimate of HR_{max}. A more accurate equation is $HR_{max} = 208 - (0.7 \times age)$. Compare the two equations:

Age	220 – age	208 – (0.7 × age)
20	200	194
30	190	187
40	180	180
50	170	173
60	160	166
70	150	159
80	140	152

You can see that the differences between the two equations range from 0 to 12 beats per minute (bpm) across this age range. That's not a huge numerical difference; the real difference lies in how accurately the equations predict HR_{max} in large groups of people. With that in mind, the second equation is a more accurate predictor of HR_{max}. From a practical standpoint, if you are leading a large group of exercisers and you want each person to have a sense of his or her HR_{max}, use $208 - (0.7 \times age)$ to make those estimates.

You know that a decline in HR_{max} is inevitable for everyone, and it doesn't matter if you're sedentary or highly fit. But *why* does HR_{max} decline with age? The answer is not known for certain, but it seems to be that with age, the electrical properties of the heart operate more slowly and the heart becomes less sensitive to hormones such as epinephrine (adrenaline). During the aging process, stroke volume (the volume of blood pumped by each beat of the heart) also declines slightly, perhaps by 10% to 20%. Cardiac output is a product of heart rate and stroke volume (CO = HR × SV), so it should be no surprise that cardiac output declines with age. And that's not all. Because cardiac output is a major determinant of $\dot{V}O_{2max}$, $\dot{V}O_{2max}$ also declines with age.

rest, when the need for O_2 is low and fat is being oxidized to produce ATP, the RER value is low, which reflects a reliance on fat oxidation for ATP production. During intense exercise, when muscles are oxidizing mostly carbohydrate to produce ATP, the RER is higher. The RER value simply reflects the ratio between fat and carbohydrate oxidation.

Oxygen deficit is another term important to understand. Figure 3.5 is a graph that shows oxygen uptake during and after intense exercise.

As the graph shows, metabolic rate remains elevated for hours after stopping exercise. This response is referred to as *excess postexercise oxygen consumption*, or EPOC. The term *oxygen debt* describes the same response, but EPOC is now the preferred term. There are many reasons why oxygen consumption remains elevated after exercise, especially after strenuous exercise: (1) it takes a few minutes for breathing and heart rate to return to resting levels, (2) body temperature stays high for a while, (3) stress hormones such as epinephrine (adrenaline) and norepinephrine are elevated, and (4) ATP and PCr stores have to be replenished, as do hemoglobin and myoglobin stores of oxygen. For all those reasons and more, oxygen consumption remains above normal resting level for minutes or sometimes hours after a workout. The longer and harder you exercise, the longer the elevation in EPOC (and in metabolic rate and calories burned).

You now have at least a basic understanding of $\dot{V}O_{2max}$, but you may have also heard of $\dot{V}O_{2peak}$ and wondered about the difference between the two. It's really pretty simple. $\dot{V}O_{2max}$ describes *maximal* oxygen consumption, typically measured during running, when virtually all muscle groups are active and using oxygen. $\dot{V}O_{2peak}$ refers to the highest oxygen consumption measured during a specific exercise. For example, in cycling the legs are very active, but the upper body musculature is less active. As a result, maximal oxygen consumption is lower compared to running, but may still be at its peak for that activity. This is a bit of scientific hair splitting, but it's helpful to know the difference between the two terms when clients, athletes, coaches, or students ask.

> The heart rate increases during exercise because of changes in nerve input to the heart's pacemaker cells. Once exercise stops, the nerve input slowly decreases and so does the heart rate.

2 Because it takes your body a few minutes to gear up all the systems needed to increase aerobic ATP production, muscles rely on anaerobic ATP production by the phosphocreatine and glycolytic systems, creating an O_2 deficit. This corresponds to the heavy breathing and excess strain you feel right at the beginning of exercise.

3 *Oxygen deficit* refers to how much oxygen would have been used if the aerobic system were able to produce all the ATP from the very second that exercise began.

4 Once your aerobic energy system is up and running, your muscles rely less on the anaerobic systems. You settle in and feel like your body has responded to the exercise intensity.

1 Whenever you begin any physical activity, your muscles have to suddenly increase ATP production from a very low level at rest to a much higher level during exercise.

5 When you stop a bout of exercise, your oxygen consumption (metabolic rate) remains elevated even though you're no longer producing ATP at a high rate. In fact, oxygen consumption can remain above normal resting values for many hours after exercise.

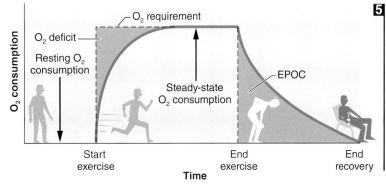

FIGURE 3.5 The oxygen deficit refers to how much oxygen would be needed to cover ATP production at the start of exercise. EPOC is the excess oxygen consumption after exercise has ended.

Adapted by permission from W.L. Kenney, J.H. Wilmore, and D.L. Costill, *Physiology of Sport and Exercise*, 7th ed. (Champaign, IL: Human Kinetics, 2020), 131.

How Does Training Help the Body Use More Oxygen?

Chapter 1 contains a list of many of the adaptations that occur with aerobic (endurance) training. Most of those adaptations are related to increasing the body's capacity to use oxygen. For instance, aerobic training stimulates muscle cells to increase their mitochondrial content as well as the enzymes associated with the Krebs cycle and the electron transport chain. To take full advantage of those adaptations, the body also has to be able to deliver more oxygen to muscle cells. That's accomplished by adaptations in the cardiovascular system. Two critical adaptations are (1) an increase in cardiac output and (2) an increase in muscle blood flow. In fact, increased cardiac output makes the greatest total contribution to increasing $\dot{V}O_{2max}$.

Recall that cardiac output is determined by heart rate and stroke volume ($CO = HR \times SV$). Although training does not alter maximum heart rate, training does increase stroke volume (the volume of blood pumped with each beat of the heart). Stroke volume increases with training because the heart's left ventricle becomes a larger and stronger pump, pushing out more blood with each beat. Blood volume (the total amount of blood in the body) also increases with training, further helping the heart to increase its output. If you've studied exercise physiology, you might remember the *Fick equation*: $\dot{V}O_2 = CO \times a\text{-}\bar{v}O_{2diff}$. In simple terms, this equation states that $\dot{V}O_2$ increases whenever cardiac output and oxygen extraction increase. (The a-$\bar{v}O_{2diff}$ refers to the difference between the oxygen content of blood in arteries and in veins; a larger value means that more oxygen has been extracted and used.)

During an exercise bout, the body must make many adjustments to ensure that all cells receive an adequate supply of blood, oxygen, and nutrients. Because active muscle cells need more blood, oxygen, and nutrients than less active cells, the body makes the necessary adjustments. Follow the steps shown in figure 3.6 for a summary of the key adjustments that occur in the cardiovascular system during exercise.

Blood volume decreases during vigorous exercise for three reasons: (1) some blood plasma is pushed out of the vessels as the result of the increase in blood pressure, (2) some plasma is drawn from the vessels into muscle cells in response to osmotic forces, and (3) some plasma water is lost as sweat. To cope with the decrease in blood volume that naturally occurs during exercise, heart rate increases to help maintain cardiac output.

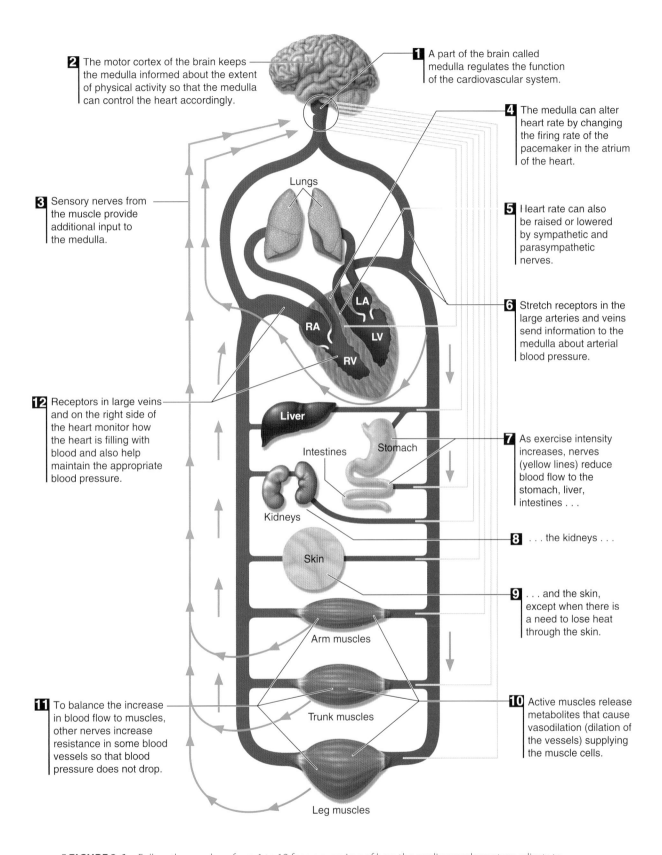

2 The motor cortex of the brain keeps the medulla informed about the extent of physical activity so that the medulla can control the heart accordingly.

1 A part of the brain called medulla regulates the function of the cardiovascular system.

4 The medulla can alter heart rate by changing the firing rate of the pacemaker in the atrium of the heart.

3 Sensory nerves from the muscle provide additional input to the medulla.

5 Heart rate can also be raised or lowered by sympathetic and parasympathetic nerves.

6 Stretch receptors in the large arteries and veins send information to the medulla about arterial blood pressure.

12 Receptors in large veins and on the right side of the heart monitor how the heart is filling with blood and also help maintain the appropriate blood pressure.

7 As exercise intensity increases, nerves (yellow lines) reduce blood flow to the stomach, liver, intestines . . .

8 . . . the kidneys . . .

9 . . . and the skin, except when there is a need to lose heat through the skin.

11 To balance the increase in blood flow to muscles, other nerves increase resistance in some blood vessels so that blood pressure does not drop.

10 Active muscles release metabolites that cause vasodilation (dilation of the vessels) supplying the muscle cells.

Lungs

LA
RA
LV
RV

Liver
Stomach
Intestines
Kidneys
Skin
Arm muscles
Trunk muscles
Leg muscles

FIGURE 3.6 Follow the numbers from 1 to 12 for an overview of how the cardiovascular system adjusts to exercise to ensure that adequate blood, oxygen, and nutrients are delivered to active muscles.

Reprinted by permission from L.W. Kenney, J.H. Wilmore, and D.L. Costill, *Physiology of Sport and Exercise*, 7th edition. (Champaign, IL: Human Kinetics, 2020), 213; Adapted Coyle (1991).

One of the many benefits of regular exercise is maintenance of healthy blood pressure. High blood pressure (hypertension) is associated with increased risk of heart attack and stroke, which is why doctors and nurses check the blood pressure of patients during every office visit. The average "normal" blood pressure is 120/80. These numbers are just shorthand to indicate that the blood pressure is 120 mmHg (millimeters of mercury is a unit that depicts pressure) in the large arteries (such as in the upper arm, where the blood pressure cuff is placed) and 80 mmHg between heartbeats, when the heart is at rest. The higher number is referred to as systolic pressure; the lower number is diastolic pressure. During exercise, systolic pressure rises as exercise intensity increases. Diastolic pressure remains the same or may even drop a bit. Improving fitness does not alter resting blood pressure in healthy people but can reduce both systolic and diastolic pressures by 6 to 7 mmHg in people with hypertension.

What Limits Aerobic Endurance Capacity?

If you train smart and hard, why can't you continue to improve your $\dot{V}O_{2max}$? It turns out that the major limit to aerobic capacity has to do with oxygen delivery to active muscles. Muscles of fit endurance athletes have enough mitochondria and oxidative enzymes to easily handle the oxygen delivered in the bloodstream. In fact, endurance performance is improved when exercisers breathe air enriched with oxygen, showing that muscles are capable of using more oxygen than what is normally delivered to them. The supply of oxygen to muscles limits aerobic capacity. In other words, the upper limits of cardiac output and muscle blood flow establish a top end for aerobic capacity ($\dot{V}O_{2max}$).

Even though being out of breath is always associated with hard exercise, breathing does not limit performance in healthy exercisers. That means that the lungs are capable of supplying as much oxygen as muscles can handle, but the muscles reach their maximal capacity to use the oxygen before the lungs reach their limit to deliver oxygen into the blood.

Improving Aerobic Capacity

If you were to create a training plan to maximize a person's aerobic capacity, what should be the length of the training program? Three months? Six months? Two years? More?

Research indicates that a person's highest attainable $\dot{V}O_{2max}$ can be achieved after roughly 12 to 18 months of proper training. Fortunately, even though $\dot{V}O_{2max}$ may hit a limit, endurance performance can continue to improve because training can increase the lactate threshold, allowing endurance athletes to maintain a faster pace.

The 12- to 18-month time frame to improve $\dot{V}O_{2max}$ is likely true for most people, but as with all physiological adaptations, some people will take considerably more time and others will take less time. This *biological variability* among people is due to a few factors. First, you won't be surprised to learn that heredity plays a major role in response to a training program, accounting for perhaps 50% of capacity to improve $\dot{V}O_{2max}$. As unfair as it may seem, some untrained people with no history of endurance training have high $\dot{V}O_{2max}$ values (e.g., >60 ml/kg/min). Lucky them.

Initial training status also affects how much $\dot{V}O_{2max}$ can increase. For example, a client who is new to fitness training has a greater potential to improve his $\dot{V}O_{2max}$ than a client who has been training for years. Both clients can achieve higher $\dot{V}O_{2max}$ values, but the untrained client will experience a larger relative improvement.

A woman's $\dot{V}O_{2max}$ value, on average, will be about 10% less than that of a man of similar age and training status. That difference may not mean much when it comes time to compete, because it's common for female runners, swimmers, cyclists, and rowers to post faster times than many men. This reality reflects individual variations among men and women and is one more example of why $\dot{V}O_{2max}$ is not a good predictor of endurance performance.

Recall from chapter 1 that some people are high responders to training while others are low responders, and that's certainly true of improvements in $\dot{V}O_{2max}$. Imagine a group of people with similar $\dot{V}O_{2max}$ values who then complete a 12-week endurance training program. Improvements in individual $\dot{V}O_{2max}$ values in response to such a training program may range from 0% to 50%. Imagine how frustrating it must be to train hard and have no improvement in $\dot{V}O_{2max}$! However, such low responders will eventually respond to training; it just takes them longer to do so.

A benefit of aerobic training is the increased production of red blood cells. But the percentage of blood volume taken up by red blood cells (known as the hematocrit) actually falls over the first couple of weeks of training because the increase in blood volume is greater than the increase in red blood cells. Hematocrit eventually returns to normal, and performance is enhanced from both the increase in blood volume and in the number of red blood cells.

Performance Nutrition Spotlight

Results of some studies suggest that certain nutrients can help lower blood pressure in hypertensive individuals. For example, foods such as spinach, celery, arugula, and beets contain nitrates, which have been shown to lower systolic blood pressure when consumed in sufficient amounts. This is another example of how diet and exercise can improve overall health.

Oxygen Delivery and Performance Enhancement

Proper training can increase oxygen delivery to active muscles by increasing cardiac output, capillary density, and maximal blood flow in active muscles. Those are the adaptations that enable improvements in endurance performance. But as some athletes have shown, there are other ways to improve oxygen delivery and endurance performance.

Prohibited Techniques

Blood doping is one illegal approach to increasing aerobic capacity. It involves removing and storing blood from an athlete, waiting a few weeks for the athlete's body to replenish the lost blood, and then infusing the stored blood into the athlete. This process results in increased oxygen delivery and improved performance. Blood doping increases blood volume and hemoglobin content so that more blood and oxygen can be delivered to active muscles. The World Anti-Doping Agency, the U.S. Anti-Doping Agency, and other sport governing bodies consider blood doping as cheating because it is a shortcut to improved performance that is not the result of training.

Another illicit way to increase oxygen delivery is with injections of *erythropoietin* (EPO). EPO is naturally produced by the kidneys to ensure a sufficient number of red blood cells in the bloodstream. EPO promotes the formation of red blood cells by bone marrow. EPO injections result in increased red blood cell production, which means increased hemoglobin and greater oxygen delivery. One risk of using EPO is that too many red blood cells can be produced, increasing the viscosity (thickness) of the blood and creating an enormous strain on the heart. It is thought that dozens of young, healthy competitive cyclists may have died of heart attacks related to their use of EPO.

Other Techniques

Some endurance athletes sleep in altitude tents or rooms with a reduced amount of oxygen in the air (lower partial pressure of oxygen, to be precise) to stimulate natural EPO production and increase the red blood cell content of their blood. Those techniques for increasing red blood cell mass are not illegal. Competitive swimmers often engage in *hypoxic training* by reducing their breathing frequency or holding their breath during repeat swims. Elite distance runners may spend time at altitude to try to benefit from exposure to the hypoxic (lower-than-normal oxygen content) environment, a topic covered in more detail in chapter 10. The intent of hypoxic training is to induce physiological and metabolic changes that promote greater adaptations.

For athletes interested in improving muscle strength, a variation of hypoxic training is *blood flow restriction*, in which the blood flow to arms or legs is reduced during strength training to create a greater training stress. It appears that blood flow restriction can also promote positive changes that result in improved strength and muscle mass, even when training with light weights.

For most people, it does not make sense to live at altitude, sleep in altitude tents, or restrict blood flow during strength training. A simpler solution for those looking for improved performance is to alter the intensity, duration, and frequency of training to create a progressively increasing training stress.

Breathing oxygen-enriched air from a tank improves endurance performance by increasing oxygen delivery to active muscles. Even though red blood cell hemoglobin is almost always completely saturated with oxygen (about 98% of the hemoglobin in blood is saturated with oxygen), breathing 100% oxygen will increase the amount of oxygen in blood by about 10%, enough to improve endurance performance. For mountain climbers at high altitude, it makes sense to carry an oxygen tank to help ensure improved performance and safety. That's not true for athletes in any other sport except scuba diving.

What about breathing 100% oxygen during recovery, as American football players are often seen doing on the sidelines? Sport scientists have not been able to find a physiological benefit to breathing oxygen during recovery. In other words, breathing oxygen during recovery does not improve performance in a subsequent bout of exercise. This continuing practice is a good example of the *placebo effect*—when psychological expectations trump physiological benefits. For that reason alone, oxygen tanks are unlikely to disappear from football sidelines.

Eating more vegetables might actually be an effective way to improve endurance performance. Vegetables such as celery, carrots, beets, and rhubarb contain nitrates, a simple combination of one nitrogen atom linked to three oxygen atoms. In the body, nitrates are converted into the biologically active compound nitric oxide (one nitrogen and one oxygen). Research shows that increasing nitric oxide production improves muscle blood flow, reduces the oxygen cost of exercise, and improves both endurance and prolonged intermittent high-intensity performance. In other words, less oxygen is used during exercise even though the exercise intensity is unchanged. From a health standpoint, nitrate ingestion is associated with lower blood pressure, a real plus for those who struggle with hypertension.

Chapter Summary

- The oxygen in the air we breathe diffuses into the bloodstream in the lungs and is transported by red blood cells to cells throughout the body, where it is used in the electron transport chain in mitochondria to produce ATP, CO_2, H_2O, and heat.

- Red blood cells are packed with millions of hemoglobin molecules, each of which can transport four O_2 molecules attached to four iron molecules.

- As the red blood cells pass through tiny capillaries, O_2 diffuses from the blood into the nearby cells.

- Because O_2 is critical for ATP production, the volume of O_2 we can use is an important measure of aerobic fitness.

- $\dot{V}O_2$ at rest is a measure of resting metabolic rate (RMR) and is used to calculate how many Calories (kcal) we expend at rest and during physical activity.

- The oxygen deficit that occurs at the beginning of exercise and the excess postexercise oxygen consumption (EPOC) that happens after exercise are other features of oxygen consumption.

- The volume of O_2 you use is determined by your cardiac output and the volume of O_2 taken up by your cells. Both of these characteristics improve with training, accounting for the improvement in $\dot{V}O_{2max}$ and performance.

Review Questions

1. Describe how oxygen is transported from the lungs to muscle cells and how carbon dioxide is transported from muscles to the lungs.

2. Identify the percentages of nitrogen, oxygen, and carbon dioxide in the air.

3. Explain what happens to the carbon atoms in glucose and fatty acids when those molecules are completely oxidized to produce ATP molecules.

4. Describe the significance of $\dot{V}O_{2max}$ as a predictor of endurance performance.

5. Identify the components of $\dot{V}O_{2max}$ and discuss how each is altered by training.

CHAPTER FOUR

Fatigue: What Is It Good For?

Objectives:

- Discover that fatigue has many causes but also many benefits in maximizing the adaptations to exercise training.
- Recognize how and when to incorporate fatigue in a training program designed to maximize improvements in fitness and minimize the risk of overtraining.

No one likes to become fatigued, even though it's a natural consequence of hard exercise. Fatigue saps physical capacity, drains mental focus, and exhausts the desire to maintain the intensity of exercise. Fatigue is often equated with failure, especially when fatigue occurs during competition. After all, one of the most important benefits of training is to delay the onset of fatigue for as long as possible. Whether you're sprinting 100 meters or pacing yourself through a marathon, fatigue is what slows you down. *Fatigue—physical or mental—simply refers to the inability to maintain a task despite trying to continue.*

You know from personal experience that fatigue comes in various forms. The mental fatigue you encounter after a long day at work feels different from the fatigue of a long day of physical labor. The intense fatigue that accompanies a fast 400-meter run is not at all like the fatigue resulting from a marathon run. Yet, in both cases fatigue limits the ability to maintain a fast pace. The stark difference in how you sense fatigue is an indication that fatigue has various causes that are related to the intensity and duration of exercise.

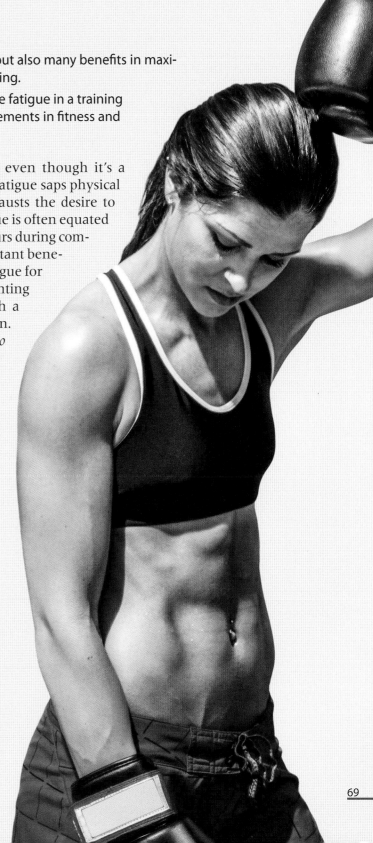

What Causes Fatigue?

Table 4.1 is a list of the mechanisms by which fatigue can occur. For example, fatigue can result from *peripheral* reasons that impair the transmission of impulses from nerve to muscle or limit the ability of muscle cells to produce ATP molecules at a rate required to maintain the desired intensity of exercise. Fatigue can also occur as the result of *central* limitations, or the inability of the brain and nervous system to maintain the neural requirements for continued exercise. Central fatigue can take the form of losing the desire or motivation to continue exercise or a decline in some aspect of the motor skills associated with continued exercise. In other words, you lose focus, become less coordinated, and either slow down (willingly or unwillingly) or stop. Some scientists suggest that central fatigue helps protect highly motivated athletes from pushing themselves too far, even beyond the point when peripheral fatigue would cause most people to stop.

During brief, all-out efforts, muscle cells are capable of increasing the rate of ATP production 1,000 times that of the rate at rest. Any factor that reduces the rate of ATP production required to sustain a certain exercise intensity will result in fatigue.

TABLE 4.1 **Possible Causes of Fatigue During Exercise**

Cause	What it means	How it limits exercise
PCr depletion	Cells run short of the phosphocreatine used to quickly generate ATP	Reduces the capacity for high-intensity contractions
ATP depletion	When ATP cannot be produced at the needed rate, ATP levels in muscle cells drop	Reduces the capacity for high-intensity contractions
Glycogen depletion	Glycogen deposits, the storage form of glucose in muscles and liver, fall to low levels	Less glucose is available for use as fuel, reducing the rate at which muscle cells can produce ATP
Hypoglycemia	Low blood sugar	Reduces the uptake and use of glucose by brain, nerves, and muscle cells, making exercise feel more difficult
Hypovolemia	Low blood volume, often due to dehydration	Reduces cardiac output, the ability of the heart to supply blood and oxygen to working muscles
Hyperthermia	High body temperature	Makes exercise feel more difficult and reduces the brain's desire to continue exercise
Metabolic acidosis	An accumulation of lactate molecules and hydrogen ions in blood and muscles	Reduces the ability of muscle cells to contract. Increases breathing rate.
Disrupted neural transmission	Temporarily impaired nerve function	Alters signals to and from muscle, negatively affecting coordination and strength
Disrupted brain activity	Temporarily impaired brain function	Reduces the desire to continue exercise and the muscular coordination required to maintain exercise

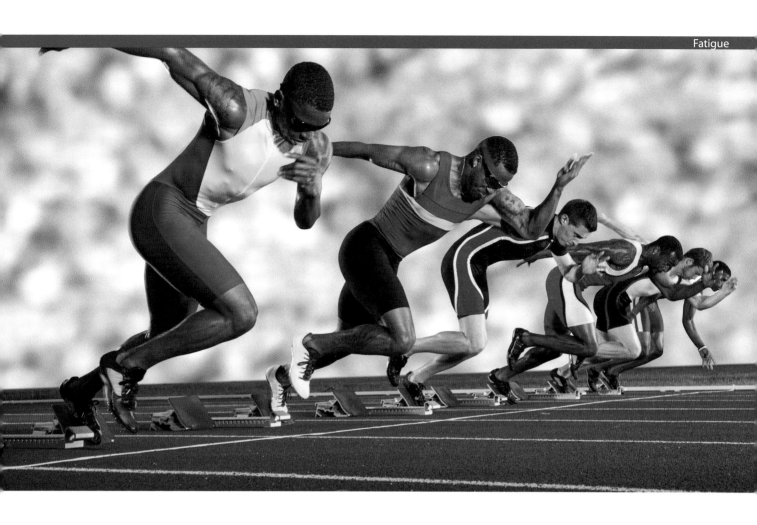

Table 4.2 contains a simple summary of peripheral and central factors in exercise fatigue. Delaying the onset of fatigue is a central feature of effective training programs. Yet, periodic fatigue during training is a primary impetus for the many adaptations that must eventually occur to keep fatigue at bay. For example, completing sets of resistance exercise to temporary failure uses fatigue as a stimulus to provoke the intracellular signals required to increase the production of contractile proteins. The temporary fatigue encountered during high-intensity interval training (HIIT) is a stimulus for increasing the buffering capacity of muscle and blood. And the fatigue felt during prolonged exercise results in mitochondrial biogenesis—the production of more ATP-producing mitochondria.

To help you understand how fatigue occurs and how training, nutrition, and hydration can help delay the onset of fatigue and improve performance, take a brief look at each cause of fatigue and its underlying mechanisms (see Table 4.1).

TABLE 4.2 **A Simplified Way of Thinking About Fatigue**

Exercise intensity	Example	Likely primary cause of fatigue	Possible secondary causes of fatigue
Moderate (below the lactate threshold)	Long hike or bike ride	Central fatigue	Dehydration, glycogen depletion, hypoglycemia
Heavy (at or just above the lactate threshold)	Marathon race	Glycogen depletion	Dehydration, central fatigue, hypoglycemia
Severe (well above the lactate threshold)	Any all-out or very high-intensity effort	Impaired ATP production due to metabolic acidosis	Hyperthermia, dehydration

Phosphocreatine and ATP Depletion

These two factors are discussed together because they are so closely related during high-intensity efforts. In figure 4.1 you'll see that at the start of all-out exercise, PCr is quickly broken down to form the ATP needed for rapid muscle contraction. Some of the ATP molecules stored inside muscle cells are also immediately used for muscle contraction. That combination of PCr and ATP is enough to maintain all-out exercise for only a few seconds, but that's long enough to allow for glycolysis to ramp up ATP production. As you can imagine, all-out exercise quickly reduces the supply of PCr in active muscle cells. ATP supplies also drop quickly but never fall as much as PCr levels because ATP is continuously produced by other pathways. Once PCr and ATP supplies fall sufficiently, the initial pace of exercise begins to slow because the rate of overall ATP production has slowed. That's why even the world's elite sprinters can maintain top speed for only about 4 seconds before they begin to slow.

It would be a waste of money to buy ATP and PCr supplements because both molecules are broken down during digestion. However, consuming creatine supplements has been shown to increase muscle PCr stores, at least in those study participants whose muscle creatine stores are not already at maximum. Creatine supplementation has also been shown to increase performance in repeated bursts of high-intensity exercise. This change may enhance the response to intense interval training by allowing more intense training sessions.

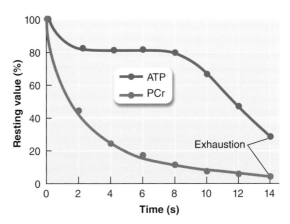

FIGURE 4.1 PCr and ATP levels fall quickly during all-out exercise.

Reprinted by permission from W.L. Kenney, J.H. Wilmore, and D.L. Costill, *Physiology of Sport and Exercise*, 7th ed. (Champaign, IL: Human Kinetics, 2020), 59

Signs of Fatigue
- Unwillingness to continue exercise
- Inability to maintain pace or intensity
- Reduced muscle strength
- Clumsy movements
- Inaccurate movements
- Muscle pain and discomfort
- Perception of increased effort required to maintain exercise

Glycogen Depletion

Whenever muscles contract, the glycogen molecules that are scattered through-out muscle cells are continuously broken down to supply most of the glucose molecules that enter glycolysis for the production of ATP. Glycogen is a critical fuel for muscles; when glycogen stores fall to low levels, exercise feels much more difficult and performance is impaired. The term *glycogen depletion* does not mean that muscle glycogen levels have fallen to zero, it simply means that glycogen stores in muscles have dropped to a critical level below which muscle cells significantly slow their use of glycogen. As a result, exercise intensity falls dramatically—the athlete has "hit the wall." The study summarized in Figure 4.2 reported that as glycogen levels fell in the gastrocnemius muscle during tread-mill running, the participant rated the exercise to be more and more difficult, even though his running speed remained unchanged. This is a good example of peripheral (glycogen depletion) and central (increased perceived exertion) factors combining to cause fatigue.

Muscle glycogen can definitely be a limiting factor during endurance exercise, but keep in mind that high-intensity exercise also relies on muscle glycogen. In fact, the rate at which muscle glycogen is broken down during sprinting can be 40 times faster than the rate during walking. You might have also noticed in figure 4.2 that during the first hour of treadmill running, muscle glycogen stores fell faster than after the first hour. Muscles are happy to break down glycogen to produce ATP and do so whenever glycogen levels are high. Later in exercise, as glycogen levels drop, muscles rely more on the oxidation of fatty acids to produce ATP, causing reduced speed or, as in the case of the person in figure 4.2, increased discomfort as exercise continues. In this example, you might say that the person hit the wall after about 1.5 hours of treadmill running, the point at which low muscle glycogen was associated with a large increase in perceived exertion.

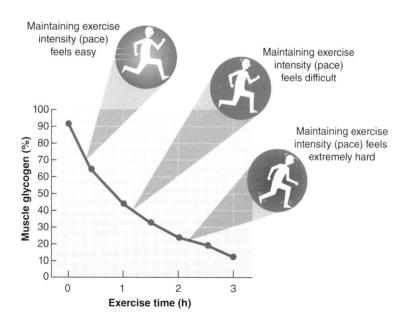

FIGURE 4.2   During prolonged exercise, muscle glycogen levels decline, exercise feels much more difficult, and pace slows.

Adapted from D.L. Costill, *Inside Running: Basics of Sports Physiology* (Indianapolis: Benchmark Press).

The intensity of exercise determines how rapidly muscle glycogen
is broken down; the more intense the exercise, the faster the rate of glycogen depletion. For this reason, anyone who trains hard should consume a diet high in carbohydrate to replace the muscle glycogen used during training. In other words, high-carbohydrate diets are not just for endurance athletes.

The type of exercise affects how muscle glycogen is used, as mentioned in chapter 1. For example, sprinters use more glycogen from their type II fibers, while endurance athletes use more glycogen from their type I fibers. Other factors can influence how active muscle cells use their muscle glycogen. For example, glycogen is depleted at different rates depending on which muscles are most stressed by a particular exercise. In figure 4.3 you'll see that running on the level, uphill, or downhill determines which muscles use the most glycogen.

If muscle glycogen is so important to performance, what is the best way to protect glycogen stores? For example, by consuming carbohydrate during exercise, can you slow the use of muscle glycogen? Unfortunately, the answer to that question seems to be no, although a few studies have reported glycogen sparing with carbohydrate feeding. Consuming a sports drink, energy bar, or carbohydrate gel can certainly improve exercise performance by helping maintain a high rate of overall carbohydrate oxidation, but overall muscle glycogen use seems to be unaffected.

Consuming carbohydrate during exercise helps maintain blood glucose levels, preventing a large drop in blood glucose, or *hypoglycemia*. During both rest and exercise, your liver has the job of adding glucose molecules to your bloodstream to maintain a normal blood sugar (glucose) level. But your liver has a supply of its own glycogen; when those limited stores are depleted, hypoglycemia occurs

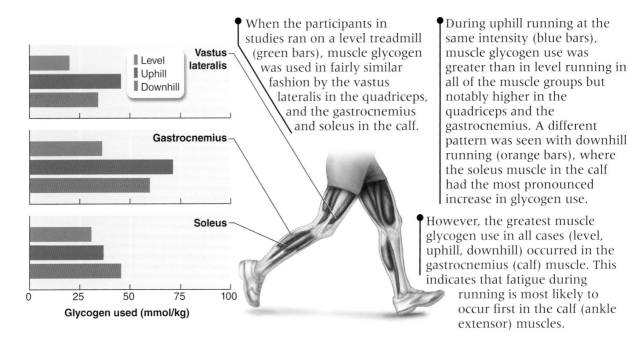

When the participants in studies ran on a level treadmill (green bars), muscle glycogen was used in fairly similar fashion by the vastus lateralis in the quadriceps, and the gastrocnemius and soleus in the calf.

During uphill running at the same intensity (blue bars), muscle glycogen use was greater than in level running in all of the muscle groups but notably higher in the quadriceps and the gastrocnemius. A different pattern was seen with downhill running (orange bars), where the soleus muscle in the calf had the most pronounced increase in glycogen use.

However, the greatest muscle glycogen use in all cases (level, uphill, downhill) occurred in the gastrocnemius (calf) muscle. This indicates that fatigue during running is most likely to occur first in the calf (ankle extensor) muscles.

FIGURE 4.3   Muscle glycogen use in three sets of leg muscles during treadmill running on the level, uphill, and downhill.
Adapted by permission from W.L. Kenney, J.H. Wilmore, and D.L. Costill, *Physiology of Sport and Exercise*, 7th ed. (Champaign, IL: Human Kinetics, 2020), 137.

unless you're able to consume carbohydrate to maintain blood glucose. One of the many reasons to recommend that athletes consume carbohydrate before beginning a morning workout is to help replenish the liver glycogen levels that dropped during sleep.

For anyone involved in hard training, muscle glycogen levels will vary widely from day to day. The goal of eating enough carbohydrate in the diet is to prevent muscle glycogen from remaining too low and impairing the ability to train hard. Large drops in muscle glycogen—as occurs in two-a-day practices—can be an important signal for adaptations required for improved fitness, as long as ample dietary carbohydrate is available to restore muscle glycogen to higher levels.

Hypoglycemia

As noted previously, when the liver runs low on glycogen, blood sugar level falls and hypoglycemia results. Symptoms include mental and physical fatigue, shakiness, weakness, and hunger. Understandably, consuming carbohydrate during exercise helps maintain a normal blood sugar level. When exhausted people who have exercised for hours without consuming carbohydrate are fed a few hundred Calories in the form of sugar, they are able to continue exercise. The reason that consuming carbohydrate has such a major impact on exercise performance is that maintaining blood glucose concentration ensures that a steady supply of glucose for ATP production is available not only for active muscles but also for the brain and nerves. The central nervous system is an obligatory user of glucose for ATP production. In other words, under normal circumstances, glucose is the only fuel used by the brain and nerves. That's why hypoglycemia can quickly cause fatigue and irritability.

Performance Nutrition Spotlight

Research shows that simply rinsing your mouth with sugar solutions can result in improved performance, even if none of that sugar is ingested. Your brain and muscles depend upon having an ample supply of glucose to fuel muscle contractions and maintain brain function. Just the sensation of having sugar in your mouth is enough to "trick" your brain and muscles into anticipating that more glucose is on its way. Mouth rinsing can be particularly helpful during intense exercise lasting less than 45 minutes because in that time very little carbohydrate can be absorbed in the small intestine and oxidized by active muscle cells. Mouth rinsing also can be helpful during times of gastrointestinal discomfort when consuming carbohydrate foods or drinks is not possible.

Dehydration

Hypovolemia is the medical term for lower-than-normal blood volume, one of the main effects of dehydration. Most people are more familiar with the term *dehydration*, so that's the term used in this text from now on.

Sweating presents a real challenge to fluid regulation because the water molecules in sweat come from the bloodstream (*vascular fluid*), from fluid that bathes the cells (*interstitial fluid*), and from fluid inside the cells (*intracellular fluid*). If you work up a big sweat, it's easy to lose water from the body a lot faster than you're able to drink it. As a result, you become dehydrated.

Even slight dehydration (e.g., a loss of 1% of body weight, just 2 pounds [1 kg] for a 200-pound [100 kg] person) results in measurable physiological changes. As dehydration worsens, so do the effects on physiology and performance, especially in warm environments. Dehydration impairs a variety of physiological functions, making it difficult and uncomfortable to maintain exercise intensity. Many athletes and clients will be at least slightly dehydrated before they begin exercise, making fluid replacement during exercise all the more important.

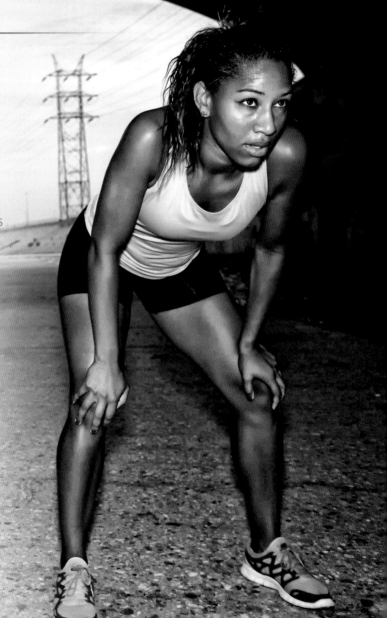

Effects of Dehydration

Increased

- Incidence of gastrointestinal discomfort
- Plasma osmolality
- Blood viscosity
- Heart rate
- Resting core temperature
- Skin temperature
- Brain temperature
- Core temperature at which sweating begins
- Core temperature at which skin blood flow increases
- Core temperature at a given $\dot{V}O_2$
- Carbohydrate oxidation
- Glycogen breakdown in muscle and liver
- Thermal discomfort

Decreased

- Blood plasma volume
- Blood flow to internal organs, including brain
- Central blood volume
- Central venous pressure
- Cardiac filling pressure
- Stroke volume
- Cardiac output
- Skin blood flow at a given core temperature
- Maximal skin blood flow
- Muscle blood flow
- Sweat rate at a given core temperature
- Maximal sweat rate
- Glycogen synthesis in muscle and liver
- Physical and mental performance

It is important to avoid dehydration, which is easily accomplished in most cases by drinking during exercise. Staying well hydrated during physical activity helps you get the most out of your body, makes exercise more comfortable, and decreases the risk of heat illness. But how much should you drink during exercise? That question has no single answer because everyone sweats at a different rate. Some people are light sweaters (<1 L/hr) and sweat only enough to moisten the skin. Most people are average sweaters (1-2 L/hr) and some people are heavy sweaters (>2 L/hr). Figure 4.4 is a simple depiction of how widely sweating rates can vary among people.

Regardless of your rate of sweating, the goal is to drink enough during exercise to minimize loss of body weight. That's why weighing yourself before and after exercise is helpful for anyone who works up a sweat on a regular basis. Loss of greater than 2 percent of body weight indicates the need to increase fluid intake during future training sessions. A gain in body weight indicates that too much fluid has been consumed. See table 4.3 for recommendations on how to stay well hydrated.

Putting aside scientific details, here is the practical message about hydration: It's always better to be well hydrated than dehydrated. That's true for overall health and particularly true for ensuring your ability to perform optimally, both physically and mentally.

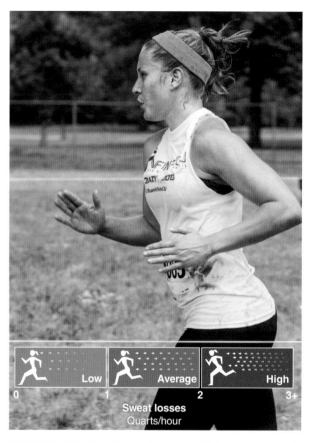

FIGURE 4.4 Sweating rates vary widely among people depending on fitness, ambient temperature, exercise intensity, genetic predisposition to sweating, and other factors.

TABLE 4.3   **Hydration Recommendations From the American College of Sports Medicine**

Before exercise	Drink 2-4 ml of fluid per lb of body weight (5-10 ml/kg BW), 2 to 4 hr before exercise to ensure euhydration (normal hydration)	Example: A 180-lb (82 kg) athlete should drink 360-720 ml (12-24 oz) of fluid in the 2-4 hr before exercise.
During exercise	Drink enough to keep loss of weight less than 2% of body weight.	Example: A 130-lb (59 kg) athlete should drink enough during exercise to weigh no less than 127.4 lb (57 kg) after exercise.
After exercise	If dehydrated, drink 125%-150% of the final fluid deficit. For example, if you are 3 lb (1.5 kg) lighter after exercise than before, drink 60-72 oz (1.8-2.1 L) to restore hydration.	Example: An athlete finishes training weighing 4 lb (1.8 kg) less than he weighed before the training session. To ensure complete rehydration, he should drink at least 80 oz (2.4 L) of fluid before the next training session.
Fluid selection	Before and after exercise, all non-alcoholic beverages can be consumed. During exercise, water and sports drinks are recommended.	

Based on T.D. Thomas et al. "Nutrition and athletic performance," *Medicine and Science in Sports and Exercise* 48, no. 3 (2016): 543-568.

Hyperthermia

One of the unavoidable effects of dehydration is an increase in core body temperature. Normal resting body temperature is 98.6 °F [37 °C; yours may be slightly lower or higher], but *hyperthermia* (when the body temperature is well above normal) can also occur in well-hydrated people either as a result of exercise in a warm environment or simply as the result of exposure to a hot environment, such as a sauna.

Body temperature naturally rises during physical activity because heat is a by-product of muscle contraction, as you learned in chapter 2. Too much of a rise in body temperature (often referred to as *core temperature*) impairs performance and increases the risk of heat illnesses such as *heat exhaustion* and *heatstroke*. A quick look at figure 4.5 confirms that even mild heat exposure impairs exercise performance. A warm environment limits the ability to exercise because as core temperature rises, muscle glycogen is broken down faster, blood is redirected to the skin to aid in heat loss, sweating rate is greater, the risk of dehydration increases, and the motivation to continue exercise lessens.

Research studies have shown that precooling muscles improves performance and preheating muscles impairs performance. That's one reason why athletes warming up for a training session or competition on a hot day should do just that—warm up, not heat up.

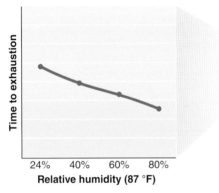

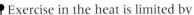

Exercise in the heat is limited by
- High core temperature
- Faster breakdown of muscle glycogen
- Blood redirected to skin instead of muscles
- Greater sweating and risk of dehydration
- Reduced motivation

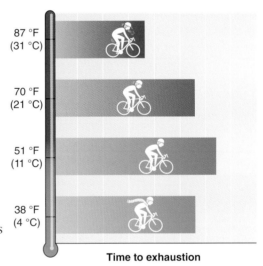

FIGURE 4.5 Heat impairs exercise performance. Studies show that at higher temperature and humidity, run times to exhaustion are reduced.

Part a data from S.D.R. Galloway and R.J. Maughan, "Effects of Ambient Temperature on the Capacity to Perform Prolonged Cycle Exercise in Man," *Medicine and Science in Sports and Exercise* 29 (1997): 1240-1249; part b data from R.J. Maughan et al., "Influence of Relative Humidity on Prolonged Exercise Capacity in a Warm Environment," *European Journal of Applied Physiology* 112 (2012): 2313-2321.

Hyperthermia is bad news for performance because a hot body—and a hot brain—don't function optimally. In fact, high body temperature limits the capacity and desire for exercise by negatively affecting the function of the cardiovascular system, muscles, and brain. As you heat up, your heart has to pump more blood to your skin to aid in heat loss, reducing blood flow to muscles, especially when you allow yourself to dehydrate. Heat also saps the brain's desire to continue exercise, causing most people to slow or stop as a way to reduce heat production and prevent heat illness. Staying well hydrated and using strategies to reduce heat gain during exercise—such as taking advantage of the wind and shade, removing some clothing, and reducing exercise intensity—can prevent hyperthermia and its negative impact on performance.

Performance Nutrition Spotlight

On very hot days, consuming cold drinks or ice-slushy drinks before exercise can aid hydration and help keep body temperature from climbing too high too fast.

Precooling Aids Performance

Getting too hot impairs performance, and getting too cold does likewise, especially for sprinters or anyone preparing for short bursts of effort. Keeping core temperature from climbing too high too fast can benefit performance by preventing hyperthermia from becoming a factor in fatigue. Staying well hydrated during exercise in the heat is one way to accomplish that, and becoming acclimated to the heat is another. So is precooling the body before intense exercise. Core temperature can be lowered slightly by consuming ice-slushy drinks, wearing a cooling vest, or sitting in cold water or a cold room. Beginning intense exercise cooler than normal increases the time it takes for core temperature to climb to levels that can impair performance.

Research shows that precooling can improve performance, especially with prolonged exercise in warm environments, when high body temperature can adversely affect the mental desire and physical capacity to continue intense exercise. It is clear that precooling strategies have to be adjusted to the conditions of training and competition that vary greatly among sports, but precooling is a strategy worth considering for anyone—athlete, soldier, or worker—who is physically active in hot environments. For example, precooling is contraindicated for sprinters for whom hyperthermia in competition is rarely an issue.

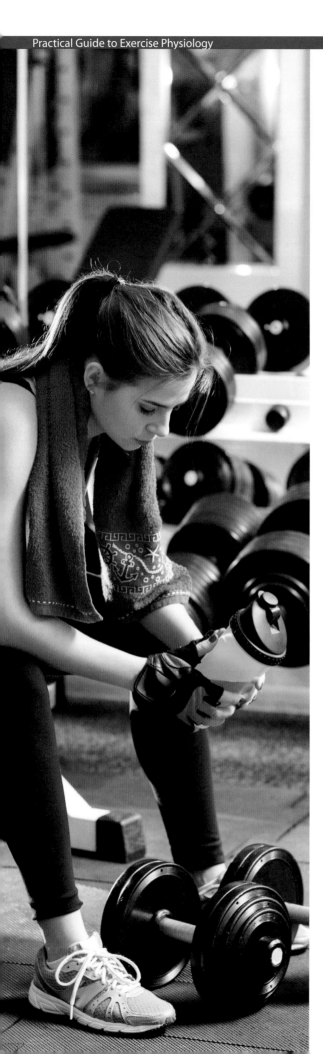

Metabolic Acidosis

You know from experience that you can't maintain intense exercise very long before it becomes so uncomfortable you are forced to slow down. That type of fatigue is often blamed on the buildup of lactic acid, but that blame is only partially accurate. Intense exercise does generate a lot of lactic acid as a by-product of the production of ATP through anaerobic glycolysis. In fact, when lactic acid rapidly accumulates inside muscle cells, it *dissociates* (breaks apart) into a lactate molecule and a hydrogen ion (H^+). In both nearby (muscle) and distant (heart and liver) cells, lactate molecules can be converted back into pyruvate molecules and enter the citric acid cycle to help produce ATP.

Lactic acid itself does not cause fatigue, but the hydrogen ions produced along with lactic acid cause muscle cells to become acidic, interfering with energy production and muscle contraction.

FIGURE 4.6 The effect of buffering systems on muscle pH. A pH of 1.5 is extremely acidic—battery acid pH is 1.0 or below, and gastric juices (stomach acid) are 1.5 to 3.0.

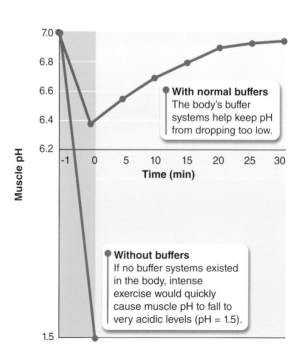

With normal buffers
The body's buffer systems help keep pH from dropping too low.

Without buffers
If no buffer systems existed in the body, intense exercise would quickly cause muscle pH to fall to very acidic levels (pH = 1.5).

It is easy to think of lactate as a garbage molecule, a nuisance by-product of metabolism that causes fatigue. Nothing could be further from the truth. Not only is lactate important in ATP production, lactate also plays a role in controlling inflammation, wound healing, and memory formation. It is estimated that you will produce about 5 ounces (148 ml) of lactic acid every day, even if you don't exercise!

When it comes to fatigue, the H^+ ion is the real troublemaker, not the lactate molecule. As H^+ ions accumulate inside muscle cells, the pH of the cell rapidly drops. In other words, the cell becomes more acidic and that reduces the cell's ability to produce ATP from glycolysis. Fortunately, muscle cells contain buffer systems that prevent pH from dropping so low that it damages the cell (figure 4.6). But the slight acidification that does occur limits the ability to continue intense exercise because low pH hampers ATP production and muscle contraction. Reduced blood flow to active muscle cells—as can occur with dehydration—can also contribute to fatigue by reducing the delivery of oxygen and glucose and slowing the removal of metabolic acids and heat.

One of the ways that a drop in muscle cell pH impairs performance is thought to be interference with how calcium ions (Ca^{2+}) function in the contractile process (figure 4.7). Recall from chapter 1 that muscle contraction depends on the release of Ca^{2+} ions from the sarcoplasmic reticulum, followed by the equally rapid uptake of Ca^{2+} ions back into the sarcoplasmic reticulum. If either of those processes is disrupted, muscle force production will decrease. Such a drop in force production (strength) is the hallmark of fatigue.

What can be done to counter metabolic acidosis during exercise? Proper training accomplishes that by increasing the buffering capacity of muscle, lessening the impact of metabolic acidosis. Some studies have reported that people can increase their capacity for intense exercise by consuming solutions containing sodium bicarbonate or sodium citrate. Both bicarbonate and citrate act as buffers to counteract the accumulation of H^+ ions that slow glycolysis and interfere with muscle contractions.

Normal process
The job of Ca^{2+} ions is to bind to troponin, causing tropomyosin strands to move just enough to uncover the active sites on the actin filaments to which myosin heads can bind and cause contraction.

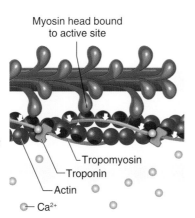

Myosin head bound to active site

Tropomyosin
Troponin
Actin
Ca^{2+}

Interference of hydrogen ions
The accumulation of H+ ions interferes with the function of Ca2+ ions, which causes a decrease in contractile force and fatigue (the inability to maintain a task).

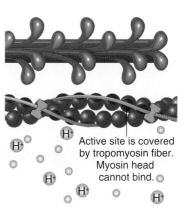

Active site is covered by tropomyosin fiber. Myosin head cannot bind.

FIGURE 4.7 Anything that interferes with how Ca^{2+} ions move in and out of the sarcoplasmic reticulum and interact with troponin will cause a reduction in muscle force production—fatigue.

Disrupted Neural Transmission

The brain, spine, and *neuromuscular junction* (where motor nerves connect to muscle) are all locations where various factors might contribute to fatigue, as depicted in figure 4.8. For example, to sustain force production during demanding exercise, motor units that were active from the beginning of the activity may drop out and previously inactive motor units will become active. This substitution of one motor unit for another can help maintain force production until such time when too many motor units either drop out or their firing rates slow to the point that force production cannot be maintained.

The brain is the control center for all voluntary human movements, and this *central drive* to continue exercise can be influenced in positive or negative ways to alter fatigue. The current thinking is that during intense or prolonged exercise, the brain can reduce the drive (desire) to continue exercise as a way to protect the body from injury or worse. Those protective mechanisms are usually effective but can be overridden by drugs such as amphetamines and by mental distractions. For example, shouting, music, and even verbal encouragement can temporarily increase the strength of muscle contractions, even in muscles that have been fatigued by prior exercise. It's also possible that a highly motivated but very fatigued athlete can continue to push so hard that hyperthermia can have life-threatening consequences. Although the brain is programmed to slow physical activity during exercise in hot weather where continuing could result in heatstroke and death, some athletes, laborers, and soldiers have ignored those symptoms with tragic consequences.

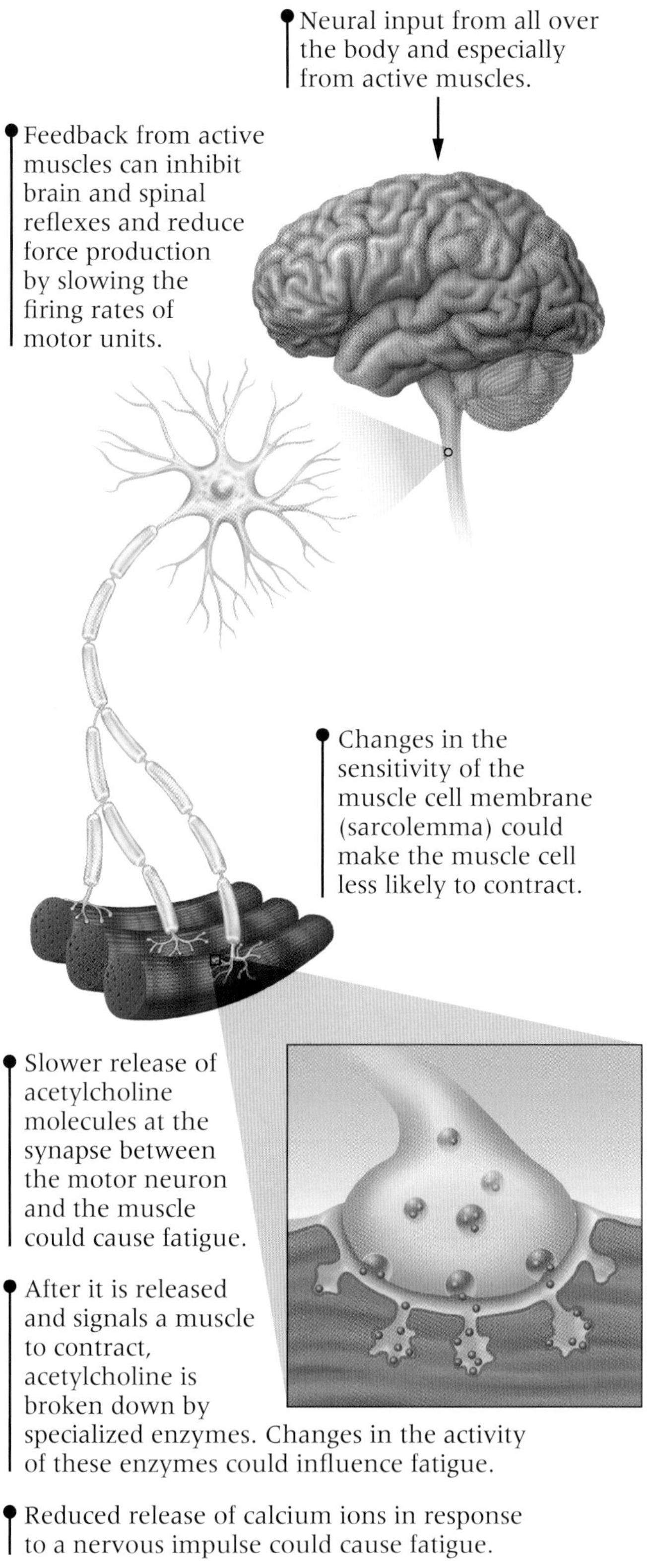

Neural input from all over the body and especially from active muscles.

Feedback from active muscles can inhibit brain and spinal reflexes and reduce force production by slowing the firing rates of motor units.

Changes in the sensitivity of the muscle cell membrane (sarcolemma) could make the muscle cell less likely to contract.

Slower release of acetylcholine molecules at the synapse between the motor neuron and the muscle could cause fatigue.

After it is released and signals a muscle to contract, acetylcholine is broken down by specialized enzymes. Changes in the activity of these enzymes could influence fatigue.

Reduced release of calcium ions in response to a nervous impulse could cause fatigue.

FIGURE 4.8 Changes in the normal operations of the brain, spinal reflexes, and neuromuscular junction can contribute to fatigue.

What's the Difference Between Fatigue and Overtraining?

Fatigue is the inability to continue a task. That could be the inability to continue to curl a dumbbell; the inability to maintain a desired pace on the track, in the pool, or on the bike; or the inability to react quickly to a stimulus. A hallmark of fatigue is that it is temporary. Within a few minutes or a few hours, depending on the exercise task, the ability to perform the task returns. In that regard, fatigue is reversible, and that rapid reversibility makes fatigue very different from overtraining.

What Is Overtraining?

Overtraining refers to physiological maladaptations and performance decrements that can last for days or weeks. Figure 4.9 shows how the normal progression for improved fitness can plateau and then either continue to improve or take a precipitous decline (overtraining). Simply put, overtraining occurs when the training stress exceeds the capacity of the athlete's body to recover and adapt.

Motivated athletes and clients are often at risk of overtraining because they tend to ignore symptoms of overtraining in their quest for greater fitness and better performance. Overtraining is a risk not just for endurance athletes. Many sports and types of fitness training, martial arts, strength training, and other physical endeavors require rigorous workouts, often more than once each day, making anyone who trains on a regular basis susceptible to *nonfunctional over-reaching* and overtraining. In contrast, periodic *functional overreaching* during a training season appears to be important in maximizing the adaptations to training.

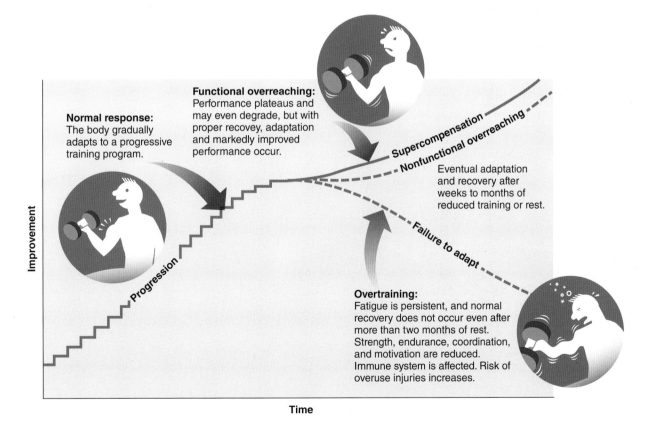

Normal response:
The body gradually adapts to a progressive training program.

Functional overreaching:
Performance plateaus and may even degrade, but with proper recovey, adaptation and markedly improved performance occur.

Supercompensation

Nonfunctional overreaching

Eventual adaptation and recovery after weeks to months of reduced training or rest.

Progression

Failure to adapt

Overtraining:
Fatigue is persistent, and normal recovery does not occur even after more than two months of rest. Strength, endurance, coordination, and motivation are reduced. Immune system is affected. Risk of overuse injuries increases.

Improvement

Time

FIGURE 4.9 Overtraining is characterized by physiological maladaptations and performance decrements that occur when the body fails to adapt to the training stimulus.

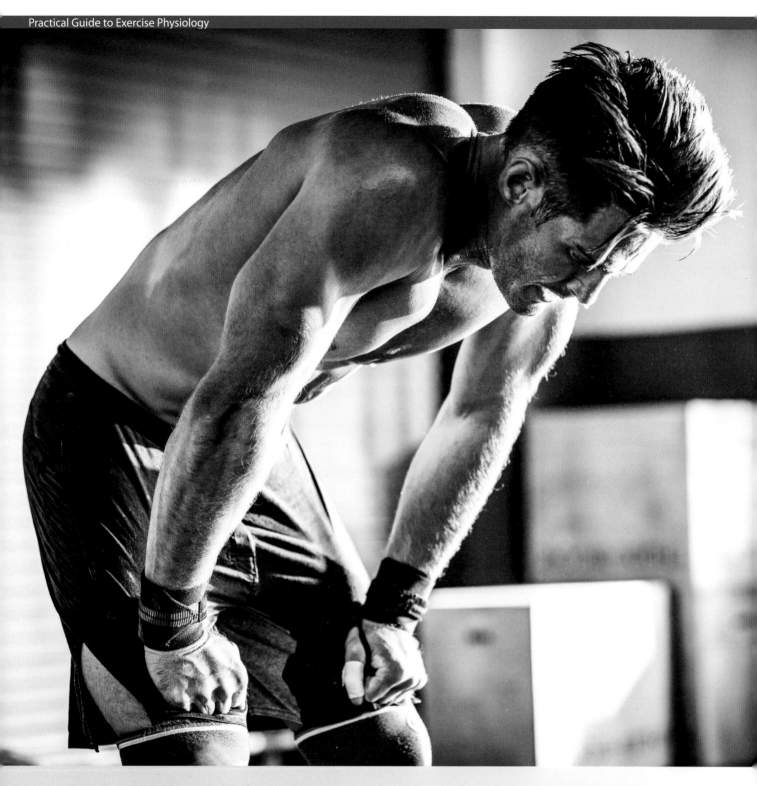

Common Symptoms of Nonfunctional Overreaching and Overtraining

- Exercise not enjoyable
- Reduced capacity for training (early fatigue)
- Loss of motivation and vigor
- Feelings of depression
- Muscle weakness
- Reduced coordination

- Achy muscles
- Loss of appetite
- Weight loss
- Sleep disturbances
- Irritability
- Inability to focus
- Resting heart rate increased or decreased

- Low heart rate variability
- Blood pressure increased or decreased
- Low energy
- Frequent colds
- Chronic muscle soreness
- Irregular menstrual cycles
- Frequent overuse injuries
- Training feels more difficult
- Performance worsens

What Role Does Fatigue Play in Adaptations to Training?

Legendary football coach Vince Lombardi was quoted as saying, "Fatigue makes cowards of us all." That may be true in some cases, but it is also true that fatigue can make better athletes of us all. It is obvious that the human body is well equipped to adapt to the stress of physical training. It should also be obvious that the extent of those adaptations is directly related to the extent of the physical stress. For example, if someone new to exercise begins a strength training program, the total extent of strength gains will depend on the total extent of the training stress. In other words, if the person trains three days each week for six months and lifts progressively heavier weights over that time, that person's strength gains will be greater than that of someone who trains just once each week and does not have much of an increase in training resistance. The overall stress of training is vastly different, so it is no surprise that the overall extent of adaptations will be different.

An obvious indicator of overall stress is the presence or absence of fatigue as a training stimulus. Not the kind of all-day, persistent fatigue that is associated with overtraining, but the periodic fatigue that occurs within training sessions. And not within every training session, but perhaps two times each week for someone training six days per week. Each time you fatigue—whether it's an individual muscle group during strength training or the entire body during endurance training—muscle cells are exposed to hundreds of intracellular signals that result in increased protein production over the next days. Those proteins can be the contractile proteins required for increasing strength and mass, the mitochondrial proteins needed for greater endurance, or the structural proteins used to make muscles and connective tissues more resistant to injury.

Fatigue during exercise maximizes adaptive responses because periodic fatigue maximizes the intracellular signals required to promote those responses. However, fatigue that occurs too often sets the stage for overtraining. Adaptations take time, which is why successful coaches understand that they cannot push their athletes hard every day; reducing training stress for a day or two after a particularly intense workout allows time for adaptations (and repair) to occur, enabling athletes to gradually and progressively increase the training stress. Ample rest, sleep, hydration, and nutrition are also required for optimal adaptations.

Effective coaching is an art guided by science.

Performance Nutrition Spotlight

Although consuming small amounts of carbohydrate during exercise may not spare muscle glycogen, doing so can prevent hypoglycemia. This practice can be helpful to all athletes during hard training and particularly to diabetic athletes who often struggle to maintain normal blood sugar levels during exercise. Consuming as little as 25 grams (100 kcal) of carbohydrate per hour can prevent hypoglycemia, although more carbohydrate (30-60 g per hr) can help improve performance.

What Causes Overtraining?

Excessive training stresses the body beyond its capacity to adapt, often with many other stressors raising the risk of overtraining. The emotional demands of balancing training with work or school; the anxiety associated with competition; fear of failure; and the stress of meeting the expectations of coaches, teammates, and parents all add to the risk of overtraining. Everyone has a unique capacity to deal with physical and emotional stress, so it's no surprise that some athletes will thrive while others fall prey to overtraining, even when they all are exposed to the same amount and type of training. That diversity in response makes it difficult to predict who is susceptible to overtraining. A coach and an athlete often don't realize that the athlete has pushed too hard for too long until it is too late.

Scientists have yet to discover a reliable marker that can be used to predict overtraining, but monitoring heart rate during exercise seems to be a useful approach. Figure 4.10 shows how exercise heart rate during a standardized exercise task fell as a result of training. That decline in exercise heart rate is exactly what is to be expected as a result of a well-designed training program. In this example, when the athlete became overtrained (OT), his exercise heart rate was 15 to 20 beats per minute *higher* than normal, an indication that his body was struggling to adapt to the stress of training.

There is also some scientific support for keeping track of an athlete's *heart rate variability* (HRV) at rest as a way to prevent overtraining. HRV is simply a measure of the time between each heartbeat and is thought to reflect changes in the health of the *autonomic nervous system* that controls heart rate, digestion, breathing, and other functions. HRV is normally high; in other words, it is normal to have considerable variability in the time between heart beats. Low HRV—when the time between heart beats is fairly consistent—is thought to indicate an overly stressful state.

As mentioned earlier in this chapter, the term functional overreaching is used to describe an important characteristic of training program design. It's important to remember that functional overreaching is very different from overtraining. Coaches and personal trainers realize that the greatest gains in strength and fitness come from training programs that require athletes and clients to regularly push themselves to temporary fatigue (overload). Done correctly, this type of training results in large gains in fitness. Done incorrectly, too much fatigue overload leads to nonfunctional overreaching and overtraining. An important part of the art of coaching—a skill that requires years to develop—is knowing when and how hard to push athletes and when to back off and allow them to rest.

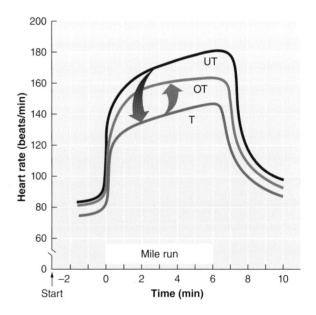

FIGURE 4.10 In overtrained people (OT), heart rate during exercise is higher than normal (T). UT is the heart rate response when the same person is untrained.

Reprinted by permission from W.L. Kenney, J.H. Wilmore, and D.L. Costill, *Physiology of Sport and Exercise*, 7th ed. (Champaign, IL: Human Kinetics, 2020), 367.

Chapter Summary

- Fatigue during all types of training helps stimulate adaptations that eventually improve fitness.
- Large drops in muscle glycogen content may cause fatigue but are also important during training as signals that cause muscle to adapt by storing more glycogen and promoting other changes that improve fitness in both endurance and stop-and-go sports.
- Fatigue—the inability to maintain a task—can be caused by many factors including PCr and ATP depletion, low glycogen stores, hypoglycemia, dehydration, hyperthermia, metabolic acidosis, and disrupted function of the central nervous system.
- Effective training causes temporary muscle fatigue on a regular basis and modestly prolonged fatigue on a periodic basis (functional overreaching) while avoiding fatigue and performance decrements that last for weeks; (nonfunctional overreaching) or months (overtraining).
- Altering muscle glycogen stores through diet and exercise can amplify the intracellular signals that promote adaptations in glycogen storage, carbohydrate oxidation, fat oxidation, mitochondrial biogenesis, and angiogenesis.

Review Questions

1. Define fatigue and describe its possible benefits.
2. Identify three possible causes of fatigue during prolonged exercise.
3. Explain how glycogen depletion is both a possible cause of fatigue and a benefit to training adaptation.
4. Describe the difference between functional and nonfunctional overreaching.
5. Discuss the differences between central and peripheral fatigue.

PART II

The Science of Training Program Design

CHAPTER FIVE

Principles of Designing Training Programs

Objectives:

- Learn the five tried-and-true scientific principles for designing training programs.
- Understand how to apply the five principles of training program design to meet individual needs, interests, and goals.

How hard, how long, and how often should people exercise to achieve their fitness goals? Common sense and science indicate that there is not one simple answer to that question because so many other factors have to be considered in the design of effective training programs. What are the person's goals and expectations? Are those goals related to improved sport performance or other objectives such as weight loss, improved cardiovascular health, or increased muscle mass? When are those goals to be achieved? In two months? Six months? A year? How much time each week can the person devote to training? How old is the person? How experienced? The answers to these and other questions are fundamental to the design of a training program because they determine the expectations and limitations around which a training program is built.

Training programs that are too difficult expose athletes and personal training clients to injury, mental and physical burnout, and overtraining syndrome. If the stress of training is not difficult enough, optimal adaptations do not occur and goals are not achieved. Training programs that are too rigid don't allow for innate differences among people to be taken into consideration. The balance between the right amount of exercise needed to optimize adaptations and too much or too little exercise varies widely among people.

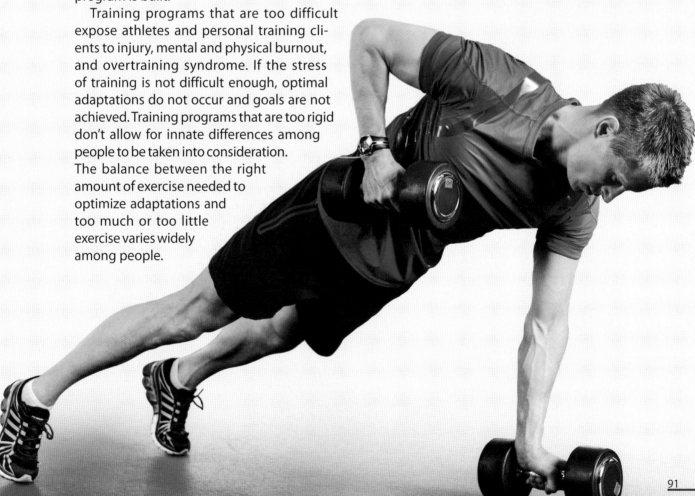

What Are the Basics of Training Program Design?

No matter the goal of the training program—speed, endurance, agility, strength, power, muscle mass, weight loss—you must consider the five principles of training program design: individuality, specificity, reversibility, progressive overload, and variation. These five scientific principles form the framework for the design of successful training programs.

Performance Nutrition Spotlight

1950s fitness guru Jack LaLanne once said that "Exercise is King and Nutrition is Queen. Put them together and you have a Kingdom." For that simple reason, every training program should have a nutrition component designed to optimize the adaptations to training.

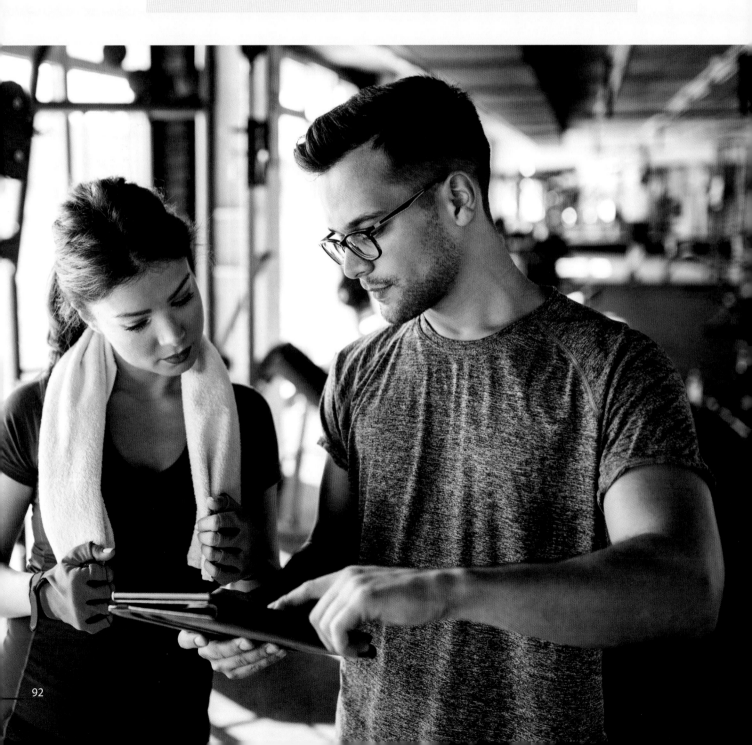

Individuality

The *principle of individuality* reflects innate differences in the ability to adapt to the stress of exercise. As illustrated in figure 5.1, some people adapt quickly, others slowly, to the same training. In other words, the same training stimulus provokes different amounts and rates of adaptation in different people. As noted in chapter 1, the differences in the adaptive response are largely genetic—some people adapt quickly (high responders), others slowly (low responders). Each person's genetic profile helps determine the starting point and the ending point. When designing programs for individuals, their unique characteristics have to be taken into account to maximize their adaptive potential through the thoughtful manipulation of exercise intensity, duration, frequency, mode, rest, nutrition, and hydration. Everyone will eventually respond to training. Low (slow) responders simply take longer or require more stimulus to improve their fitness.

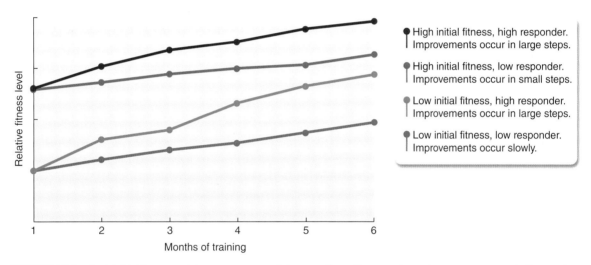

● High initial fitness, high responder.
Improvements occur in large steps.

● High initial fitness, low responder.
Improvements occur in small steps.

● Low initial fitness, high responder.
Improvements occur in large steps.

● Low initial fitness, low responder.
Improvements occur slowly.

FIGURE 5.1 Both initial fitness and the response to training are affected by genetics and vary among people. Those who design effective training programs take into consideration the fact that people begin training at different fitness levels and their progress can vary widely depending on their individual capacities to adapt to training.

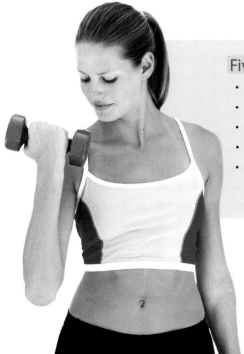

Five Principles of Program Design

- Individuality. Some people adapt quickly, others slowly, to the same training.
- Specificity. Adaptations are specific to the mode and intensity of training.
- Reversibility. Adaptations to training can be easily lost.
- Progressive overload. A gradual increase in training load prompts improvement.
- Variation (Periodization). Varying mode, duration, intensity, and frequency maximizes adaptations and reduces the risk of overtraining.

Specificity

The *principle of specificity* holds that most—but not all—training should reflect the specific demands of the sport or activity. Adaptations in muscle and other tissues are specific to the mode and intensity of training.

Common sense dictates that adaptations will be specific to the stress imposed. For instance, the adaptations that underlie increased strength and mass are best promoted by resistance training programs that stimulate the production of muscle contractile and structural proteins. For improving endurance capacity, training has to stimulate the production of mitochondrial proteins and adaptations in cardiac cells to meet the demands of prolonged exercise. Chapter 8 looks at research that shows that high-intensity interval training (HIIT) can increase anaerobic as well as aerobic power and capacity, results that lead to a slightly different interpretation of the principle of specificity. When it comes to specific activities or sports, the principle of specificity holds true: To improve performance in an activity, you should train primarily with that mode of exercise. For example, although competitive swimmers often lift weights, run, cycle, and include plyometrics and other fitness activities in their training, the majority of their training time is in the pool.

There are occasions when sport-specific training should take an initial back seat to more general training. People who are just beginning a training program—such as adults who want to participate in triathlons but have no experience in the sport—should begin with general training that creates a base fitness level on which sport-specific training can be added. This approach helps people develop fundamental training skills and reduce the risk of training-related injuries.

Eccentric training can be an important element of training specificity in many sports. Not only does eccentric training help increase muscle mass and strength, but it can also improve the muscles' ability to function as shock absorbers to help prevent landing-related injuries and cope with high external loads in sports such as soccer, skiing, ice hockey, basketball, and football.

High-Intensity Interval Training (HIIT)

For untrained and recreationally active individuals, high-intensity interval training (HIIT) can be an effective complement to traditional aerobic training. This is particularly true for people who have limited time to train or are not psychologically prepared for the demands of endurance training. Research has shown that as few as six sessions of HIIT over two weeks—a total of roughly 15 minutes of intense stationary cycling—is enough stimulus to improve exercise capacity and other markers of enhanced endurance. In one important study, HIIT was conducted three times per week for two weeks as four to six 30-second bursts of all-out cycling on a bicycle ergometer separated by 4 minutes of easy cycling. The total time devoted to training over the two-week experiment was only about 2.5 hours, with each training session involving only 2 to 3 minutes of intense exercise. HIIT improves maximal oxygen consumption and markers of cardiovascular health with a minimum commitment of time but a maximum commitment of effort. Experts suggest that endurance athletes can optimize training benefits by performing 10% to 15% of their total training as HIIT and conduct the majority of the remaining training at lower intensities to ensure that motor units needed to sustain endurance exercise are not neglected.

Reference: Gibala, M.J., & McGee, S.L. (2018) Metabolic adaptations to short-term high-intensity interval training: a little pain for a lot of gain? *Exercise and Sport Sciences Reviews.* 36(2):58-63.

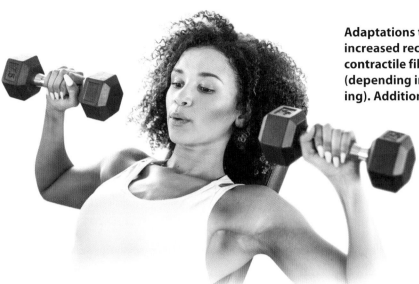

Adaptations to resistance training include increased recruitment of motor units, more contractile filaments, and greater muscle mass (depending in part on the type of resistance training). Additional adaptations are listed in chapter 6.

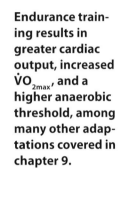

Endurance training results in greater cardiac output, increased $\dot{V}O_{2max}$, and a higher anaerobic threshold, among many other adaptations covered in chapter 9.

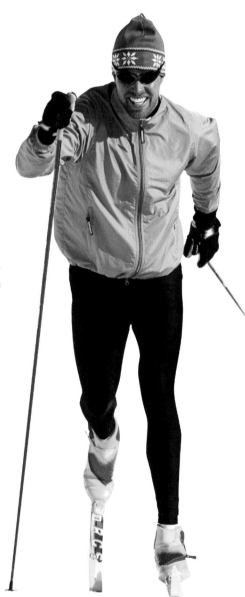

The body adapts to plyometric training with improved neuromuscular coordination, along with increased speed and power, as detailed in chapter 8.

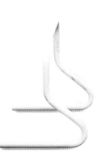

Reversibility

The *principle of reversibility* refers to the fact that the adaptations to training will be lost when training ceases or is significantly reduced.

The time and effort put into training spark adaptations in muscle, the heart, and other tissues that enable the body to tolerate increased levels of exercise intensity and duration. Those same adaptations will be lost or substantially diminished if training is reduced or discontinued (figure 5.2). However, during times of the year when it is not possible to sustain a full training program, a maintenance training program of just two days per week can preserve most of the adaptations.

"Use it or lose it" is an accurate summary of the principle of reversibility except that the saying lacks a time frame for "lose it." There is no doubt that gains in fitness are lost faster than they are achieved, but those losses can be reversed with retraining. The capacity to quickly regain strength and stamina is often incorrectly referred to as "muscle memory." It is actually the nervous system, not muscles, that retains the so-called memory that is activated by retraining.

Some scientists think that the training-induced increase in the number of nuclei within muscle cells may also impart a local memory that helps speed the return of strength after detraining. Regardless of the origin of muscle memory, the fact that retraining can stimulate fairly rapid gains in strength is important to athletes who have detrained in the offseason as well as for older adults who might repeatedly stop then restart strength training programs to help ward off *sarcopenia* (severe loss of muscle strength and mass).

A few days without training does not impair function or performance. However, injury, immobilization (e.g., casting a joint or limb), and prolonged bed rest result in rapid loss of muscle mass, strength, power, muscle endurance, flexibility, glycogen storage, and $\dot{V}O_{2max}$. In comparison, loss of fitness is considerably slower when training is stopped or reduced and the athlete or client continues other normal daily activities. In those circumstances, loss of fitness takes weeks or a few months. To maintain fitness gains, people should be encouraged to train two to three days each week using HIIT or continuous exercise at an intensity greater than 70% $\dot{V}O_{2max}$. Gains in muscle strength and in the capacity for high-intensity exercise can be maintained without training for several weeks or even months, but endurance capacity (both muscular and cardiorespiratory) declines within two weeks of detraining.

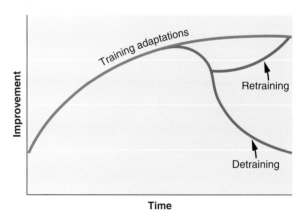

FIGURE 5.2 Detraining results in a loss of the adaptations to training, but with retraining, a trained person will adapt more quickly than an untrained person.

Progressive Overload

The *principle of progressive overload* is the cornerstone of all effective training programs. To optimize the adaptations to training, the training load (the combination of intensity, duration, frequency, and mode) should be increased in small steps to progressively overload the muscles, heart, and other tissues to gradually introduce the physical stress needed to stimulate adaptations. Virtually any type of training that stresses the body beyond the level it has become accustomed to will result in adaptations that increase the body's capacity for physical activity.

The ever-present risk is that too much training will overwhelm the body's ability to adapt and create a condition of nonfunctional overreaching or overtraining—the failure of the body to adapt, resulting in a significant reduction in training and performance capacity. In addition, overuse injuries such as shin splints and sore joints are common when the training load consistently exceeds the individual's capacity to adapt. A gradual increase in overall training load prompts the greatest improvement.

Research shows that gains in muscle strength can be maintained for at least the first three weeks of detraining before measurable losses in strength begin to occur.

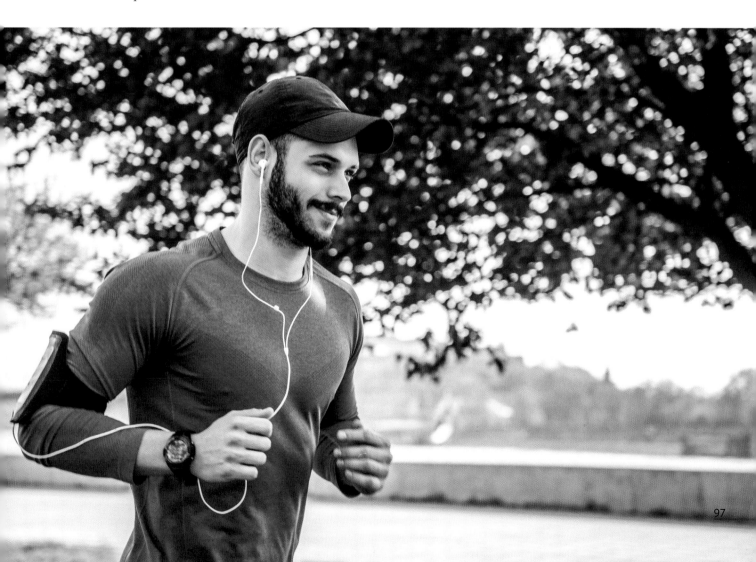

Variation (Periodization)

The *principle of variation*—also referred to as the *principle of periodization*—is the concept that purposefully varying the mode, intensity, duration, and frequency of training is effective at maintaining a training load that maximizes adaptations and minimizes the risk of overtraining.

Coaches and personal trainers recognize that repeating the same type of training over and over leads to physical and psychological staleness and is counterproductive to maximizing training adaptations. For that reason, long-term training programs should include variations that maintain an appropriate training stress while varying mode, intensity, duration, and frequency. Periodization in a training program that includes macrocycles, mesocycles, and microcycles is an example of the principle of variation. In other words, training stress is varied from day to day, week to week, and month to month to allow progressive overload to occur gradually.

Varying the mode, intensity, duration, and frequency of training is required to maximize adaptations and minimize the risk of overtraining.

Block Periodization

One reason training periodization schemes are helpful is that they require short- and long-term planning and goal setting. A challenge with periodized training is making sure the program doesn't include so many goals that the process becomes overwhelming, both physically and psychologically. Sport training (as opposed to fitness training) is particularly challenging because it requires the development of many specific skills, which complicates the design and execution of a periodized training program. An alternative approach is to include blocks of specialized training cycles that focus on just a few fitness characteristics or sport skills, creating mesocycles that build in logical order toward preestablished performance or fitness goals. In theory, block periodized training reduces the risk of overtraining that can occur as a result of trying to accomplish too much too soon. In addition, block periodization allows athletes and clients to narrow their training focus to fewer short-term goals, increasing the likelihood of noticeable improvements before moving on to the next training block.

Reference: Issurin, V.B. (2010). New horizons for the methodology and physiology of training periodization. *Sports Medicine, 40*(3):189-206.

What Makes an Effective Training Program?

Training to reach a goal would be easy if all you had to do is exercise a little harder today than you did yesterday. With each day you'd be in better shape than the day before. As long as you added more exercise stress with every passing day, your body would continually adapt and you'd get fitter and fitter. If only that were the case.

In figure 5.3, example A depicts the progress that would be made if you were able to improve every day. Example B illustrates the overtraining syndrome that usually occurs if you try to follow the pattern in example A: too much training too soon without adequate rest. Example C shows the stair-step approach of a progressive overload training program that includes periods of reduced workload, allowing the body regular opportunities to adapt to the stress of training before the training load is gradually increased.

There are many variations of periodized training programs, but all include alternating periods of increased and decreased workload. These cycles stress the body for a period of time (the stimulus) and then allow time for adaptations to occur (the response). As illustrated in the following equation, throughout each cycle, it is essential to build in ample rest, sleep, nutrition, and hydration (the facilitators) to optimize the desired adaptations and reduce the risk of overtraining.

Stimulus	**+**	**Facilitation**	**=**	**Response**
Proper training		Nutrition		Faster
		Hydration		Stronger
		Rest		More powerful
		Sleep		More flexible

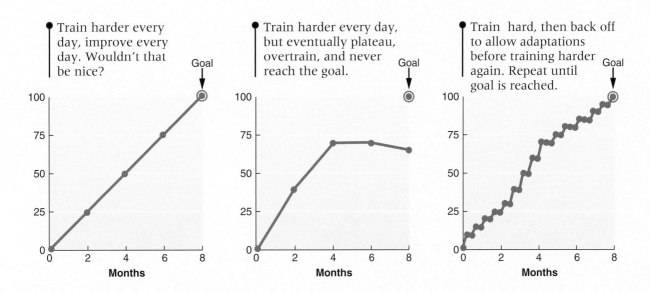

FIGURE 5.3 Three hypothetical examples of eight-month training programs illustrate how periodization can help ensure that goals are reached.

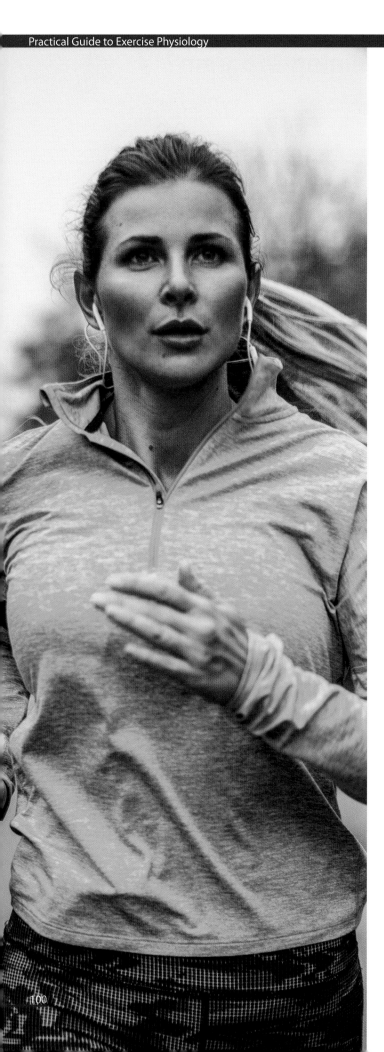

There is an endless variety of periodized training programs because each program has to take into consideration several factors. As an obvious example, a training program for football players in middle school will be quite different from a training program for college-aged football players. Likewise, a strength training program for a college-aged swimmer will be markedly different from that for a 44-year-old working mother who likes to swim for fitness. Table 5.1 summarizes the factors that have to be considered in the design of any training program. Answers to these 10 questions will help guide the creation of a training program that is tailored to meet the individual needs, interests, and goals of the athlete or client.

Adaptation Is the Goal

The word *adaptation* is used repeatedly throughout this book because the intent of training is to maximize adaptations in muscle and other tissues. To refresh your memory, all adaptations occur as a result of individual cells producing more functional proteins such as enzymes, signaling molecules, contractile proteins, and structural proteins. An increase in the functional protein content of cells increases their capacity to meet the demands of exercise. Here are three examples:

1. In liver cells, adaptations in functional proteins increase the liver's capacity to store glycogen that can be used to maintain blood glucose concentrations during exercise.

2. In skeletal muscle cells, adaptations in functional proteins increase the cell's capacity to produce ATP faster and for a longer time (among many other adaptations).

3. In cells of the blood vessels, adaptations in functional proteins enable the vessels to better dilate and constrict to meet the changing demands for blood flow that occur during exercise.

Performance Nutrition Spotlight

As with carbohydrate intake, protein intake can also be manipulated to enhance adaptations to training. Ensuring adequate protein intake after training and throughout each day maximizes muscle protein synthesis (MPS). This can be accomplished by consuming 20 to 40 grams of high-quality protein soon after training (high-quality protein contains all the essential amino acids; examples include whey, soy, meat, and eggs). In addition, spreading protein intake evenly throughout the day in meals and snacks has also been shown to enhance MPS. As an easy-to-remember rule of thumb, consuming 1 gram of protein per pound of body weight per day (about 2.2 g per kg BW per day) will provide more than enough dietary protein to meet the increased demands of the most intense training. In fact, some research indicates that even half that amount is enough to satisfy the athlete's daily need for dietary protein.

TABLE 5.1   **Questions on Program Design for Three Sample Clients**

Question	Anna	Dan	John
How old is the athlete or client?	32	26	55
What are the goals?	Complete an Olympic-distance triathlon.	Race a marathon.	Increase muscle mass and lose fat.
How much experience with sport or exercise?	Ran track for two years in high school. Periodic fitness classes in college and after graduation.	Track and cross country in high school; track scholarship in college.	Golf team in high school. Has run local road races; enjoys bicycling and lifting weights.
What are the skill levels?	Beginner in swimming and cycling. Some experience with run training and road racing.	Advanced. Ran the mile in college (4:02) and has read about marathon training programs.	Above-average and seems athletic. Has tried a lot of fitness routines.
Any injuries or health problems?	No. Had shin splints in high school track season.	None.	Periodic hip pain due to arthritis.
How committed to training?	Seems excited about trying something new and indicates that she will train on her own when needed.	Very committed. Overtraining may be a risk.	Willing to train before or after work.
What is the overall level of interest in the sport or activity?	Excited to be involved in triathlon because many of her friends are triathletes.	Would like to finish under 2:20.	Motivated by the desire to maintain strength and mass as he ages.
How competitive in both intent and skill?	Beginner in both regards. Too soon to tell if she will develop a competitive streak.	Extremely competitive. Has racing experience and knows how to train.	Competition is less important than changes in body composition and fitness.
How much time able and willing to devote to training?	Willing to train at least 3 days per week.	Willing to train 6 days each week.	Thinks he can train at least 4 days each week.
What are the deadlines for accomplishing key goals?	Sprint triathlon in 3 months. Olympic distance in 5 months.	First marathon in 4 months, next one in 6 months.	Would like to see improvements within one month to 4 weeks.

Combining Progressive Overload and Variation (More on Periodization)

Optimal adaptations in functional proteins within cells occur in response to periodically *overreaching* during training, pushing the body so that it naturally adapts to increasing levels of exercise stress. A central challenge in designing any training program is to ensure that functional overreaching does not progress into nonfunctional overreaching or overtraining. One way to accomplish that goal is to follow the principles of progressive overload and variation (periodization), as illustrated in figure 5.4.

The example in figure 5.4 shows how an eight-month training program with a specific goal (that could be a weight-loss goal, a strength-related goal, a performance goal, can be broken down into training segments, or *cycles*. In this example, two four-month *macrocycles* allow for subgoals to be established so that progress toward the ultimate goal can be assessed along the way. That same approach also applies to the two-month *mesocycles* and the two-week *microcycles*. Dividing a training program into separate parts allows each part to be designed to accomplish specific fitness goals that progressively build toward the ultimate goal. If sufficient progress is not made within a microcycle, then subsequent training can be altered to ensure that future subgoals can be met. It should be noted that training responses rarely unfold as nicely as depicted in figure 5.4. The true value of periodization may be as a conceptual approach to structuring long-term training programs to include the important aspects of

FIGURE 5.4 An example of an eight-month periodized training program that incorporates macrocycles, mesocycles, and microcycles, each of which has its own goals for exercise mode, intensity, duration, frequency, and rest.

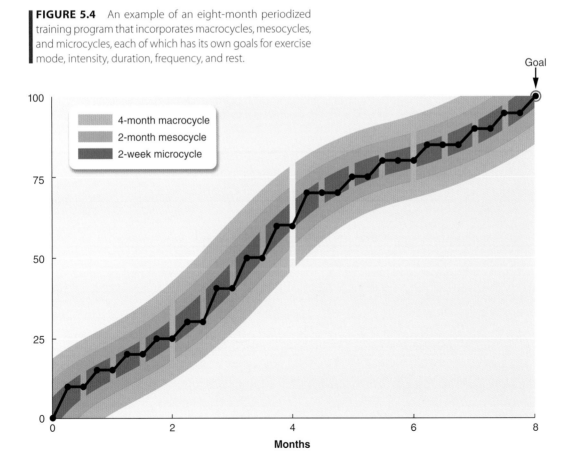

the five principles of training. For example, traditional training programs for individual sports such as running, swimming, cycling, and triathlon stress the development of an aerobic base in the early season, with emphasis on lower-intensity, longer-duration efforts. Midseason training focuses on increased intensity efforts and late-season workouts leading up to a final taper typically featuring very high-intensity work of shorter durations. Training for team sports such as football, soccer, ice hockey, volleyball, and basketball often requires heavy training early in the competitive year, supported by maintenance training once the hectic competitive season begins.

According to some research, periodized block training will provide superior results compared to traditional approaches. Instead of combining all aspects of training throughout each week, block training stresses a changing weekly or biweekly focus (microcycles) on the development of strength, endurance, power, skills, or whatever elements the coach deems important.

Notice in figure 5.4 that every increase in training capacity (the central black line) is followed by a period in which training workload plateaus (or in some cases may even decrease). Periodically lowering the training workload for a few days or even longer allows time for adaptations in functional proteins while reducing the risk of nonfunctional overreaching or overtraining. Keep in mind that figure 5.4 is simply *one* example of how the principles of progressive overload and variation (periodization) can be integrated into a training program that incorporates macro-, meso-, and microcycles.

Other variations in training program design include hard training for a certain number of days, followed by the same number of days of rest or reduced workload. Some coaches follow the 75% rule: 75% of training completed at an intensity less than 75% of maximal heart rate (HR_{max}), 15% of training at moderate intensity (e.g., 75%-85% HR_{max}), and 10% at a high intensity (e.g., >85% HR_{max}). There are countless ways to structure effective training programs. The challenge is to identify training programs that best match the needs, interests, goals, and capacities of individual athletes and clients.

Before important competitions, the training load should be gradually reduced to help maximize the various adaptations to training. This reduction in training load is commonly referred to as *tapering*. Research with swimmers, runners, and cyclists indicates that the optimal tapering strategy is accomplished over the two weeks before an important competition by decreasing the training volume by 40% to 60% without changing training intensity or frequency.

> Overtrained athletes have reductions in maximal oxygen uptake, cardiac output, systolic blood pressure, and circulating epinephrine (adrenaline) levels.

More About Overtraining

Most athletes and clients are motivated to work hard to achieve their goals. Sometimes that diligence goes too far, resulting in overtraining (also called *overtraining syndrome*). Overtraining is bad news because it can't be corrected with just a few days or even a few weeks of rest. Some athletes need six months or more of rest in order to resolve all the symptoms of overtraining, a depressing, frustrating, and trying time. With that bleak scenario in mind, you need to understand overtraining so that you can help prevent it.

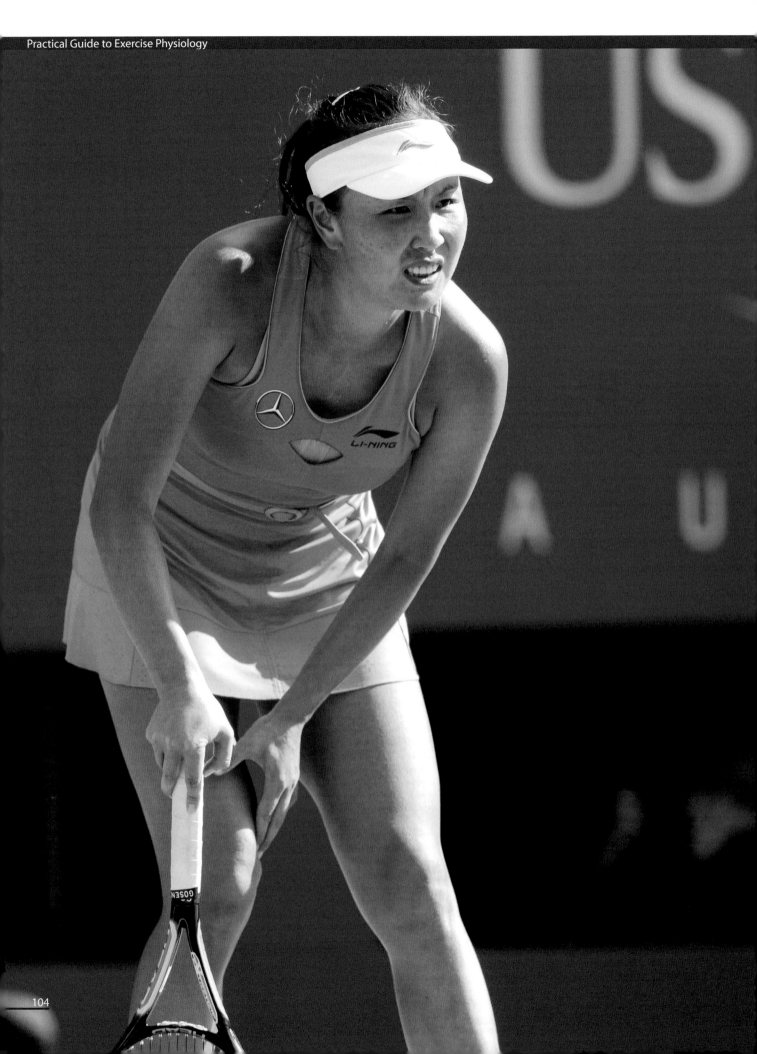

As described in chapter 4, the symptoms of overtraining include reduced strength, coordination, and endurance; loss of motivation and enjoyment; depression; loss of appetite; weight loss; sleep disturbance, irritability and lack of focus; and changes in heart rate and blood pressure. Overtraining is the result of complex interactions that occur among the nervous, endocrine, immune, and musculoskeletal systems.

Overtraining is a failure to adapt. Even worse, the athlete's performance doesn't just plateau; it deteriorates for many months and sometimes never recovers. Effective training programs are designed to produce the desired adaptations in strength, power, endurance, speed, and so on by regularly stressing muscle and other cells so that they gradually increase their capacity to withstand even greater stress. The process of stress leading to adaptation is known as *hormesis*. The various responses inside muscle cells that produce the desired adaptations can also produce negative responses (*maladaptation*) if the stress is prolonged and rest is insufficient. For example, hard training increases the temporary production of inflammatory molecules inside muscle cells that in turn promote positive adaptations within those cells. But if the training stimulus is relentless—hard training day after day—the prolonged exposure to inflammatory molecules can result in negative responses such as reduced protein synthesis, impaired immune response, loss of strength, and maladaptation of the hypothalamic-pituitary-adrenal axis, including aberrations in hormones such as prolactin and adrenocorticotropic hormone (ACTH). Unfortunately, there is no simple blood or exercise test to warn of impending overtraining. However, the good news is that periodically monitoring exercise heart rate during a standardized exercise task does seem to be an effective way to predict the possibility of overtraining (reflected by a substantially higher heart rate) and therefore the need for a few days of rest. Experienced trainers and coaches can often tell when a client or athlete begins to overtrain by noting negative changes in disposition, enthusiasm for training, and training capacity. Sometimes it is difficult to convince an athlete to back off training, but doing so may be the only way to prevent overtraining syndrome.

Some Responses to Overtraining Include Negative Alterations In

- Brain neurotransmitters
- Brain structures
- Motor nerve function
- Hormonal response
- Immune response
- Muscle function
- Body weight
- Appetite
- Sleep
- Motivation
- Energy level
- Mood
- Resting heart rate (increase or decrease)
- Resting blood pressure (increase or decrease)

Training Terms

Few things are more boring than a list of terms and their definitions, but in this case it's important that you know the pertinent terminology and meanings. For example, if an athlete asks you for advice on becoming more agile, it's essential that you both agree on the definition of *agility* so that your understanding and her expectations are clear. So, with that simple goal in mind, here are formal definitions of a few terms and some examples containing those terms.

adaptation—The process by which various changes in the body enable it to adjust to a new environment or condition. "Exercise training stimulates *adaptations* in muscle cells that improve the cells' ability to produce the energy needed for improved performance."

agility—The ability to change directions quickly and accurately. "She has really helped our team this year because her *agility* on defense has improved."

block periodization training—A training design that maintains the focus of training on a single characteristic (e.g., stamina, strength, power, skills) for a set period of time (e.g., 1 week) before the training focus changes to a different characteristic. "In the first month of the season, we rely on *block periodization training* to help our athletes establish a strong base of aerobic fitness."

detraining—The partial or complete loss of training adaptations as a result of drastically reduced training load or the complete cessation of training. "To prevent *detraining* over the Christmas break, our athletes are encouraged to do HIIT at least two days each week."

duration—The length of time in which an event occurs. "In the next training session, we'll increase your workload by increasing the *duration* of your repeat sprints."

endurance—The ability to resist fatigue, as in muscular endurance or cardiorespiratory endurance. "To improve your performance in the fourth quarter of games, you have to improve your *endurance*."

fatigue—The inability to continue a task, often associated with temporary feelings of tiredness. "For maximal muscle adaptation, it's important that you periodically exercise to *fatigue*."

functional overreaching—A planned and systematic increase in training load to stress the body beyond its normal capacity. When followed by a few days of rest or easy training it leads to improved performance capacity. "Every effective training program incorporates the concept of *functional overreaching* followed by periods of reduced training workload or rest."

hormesis—The process by which the proper stress induces positive adaptations. "Restricting blood flow to muscles during strength training is an example of using the concept of *hormesis* to enhance a training response."

intensity—The magnitude of effort. "Increasing the *intensity* of your repeat sprints will improve your anaerobic as well as your aerobic fitness."

macrocycle—A longer period of time in a training design usually encompassing many months. "We divide our training season into three *macrocycles* because that best fits our competitive schedule."

maladaptation—The body's failure to adapt to training. "Overtraining is an example of *maladaptation*, where too much training inhibits the ability of cells to properly adapt and therefore performance suffers."

mesocycle—An intermediate period of time in a training design, often just one or two months. "Our current *mesocycle* is designed to increase the number of full-court sprints our players can accomplish in a 5-minute period."

microcycle—A short period of time in a training design, usually no more than a week or two. "Our players are now in a *microcycle* where the goal is to gradually increase their bench press load by 5%."

mode—A particular form or variety of something. "We'll frequently change the *mode* of exercise to keep your mind and body from getting too accustomed to doing the same thing."

nonfunctional overreaching—Exhibiting stagnated or worsened performance that improves after a few weeks or sometimes a few months of rest or reduced training volume. "We will cut back your training load for the next three weeks to get you out of this period of *nonfunctional overreaching*."

overload—A greater-than-normal training stress or load. "For your muscles to adapt properly, you have to *overload* them gradually."

overtraining—Regularly doing more work than can be physically tolerated. "That team usually does poorly during the last part of their season because their coach doesn't understand the difference between overreaching and *overtraining*."

overtraining syndrome—Failure of the body to adapt to exercise training characterized by weeks or months of deteriorating performance and training capacity. "She has suffered from *overtraining syndrome* during each of the past two seasons because her coach insists that she train hard every day."

periodization—Division into periods. "An effective way to progressively overload the athlete's body is to use a *periodization* approach to designing the training program."

power—An index of the rate at which work can be done (power equals force times distance divided by time). Power applies similarly to athletes, racehorses, and engines. Improvements in performance often require an increase in power. "A football linebacker can increase his *power* simply by losing excess body fat and improving his speed."

repetitions (reps)—The act of repeating a function. "We'll gradually increase the number of *reps* on the bench press as you become stronger."

sets—A group of repetitions (reps). "Research shows that three *sets* of 8 to 12 reps to temporary fatigue seem to optimize gains in muscle mass."

speed—The rate of movement. In mathematical terms, speed is the distance traveled divided by the time of travel. "We can create a training program to improve your *speed* in the 40-yard sprint."

strength—The ability of a muscle to exert force. "The correct kind of resistance exercise will help older adults improve their grip *strength*, making everyday tasks easier."

tapering—Reducing the training load before important competitions in an attempt to maximize performance. "With the state championships only three weeks away, we're almost ready to start our *tapering*."

training variables—The components of a training program that can be manipulated: intensity, duration, mode, and frequency. "Our training program incorporates gradual changes in *training variables* so that our clients overreach without becoming overtrained."

training volume (or training load)—The composite of training variables. "You can increase *training volume* by increasing training frequency, duration, and intensity either individually or in combination."

work—In mathematical terms, force multiplied by distance. "You accomplish *work* whenever you walk up a flight of stairs because you raise your body weight (the force) the height of the staircase (the distance)."

workload—The amount of work expected, assigned, or accomplished. "You've really improved these last few weeks, so next week we'll increase your *workload*."

Chapter Summary

- The five core principles of training program design are individuality, specificity, reversibility, progressive overload, and variation (periodization).
- Periodization of training is the purposeful manipulation of training load (intensity, duration, frequency) and mode (endurance, speed, strength, power, etc.) over the course of the training season to optimize the adaptive responses to training.
- Improvements in fitness are lost at a faster rate than they are gained, but retraining can stimulate a fairly rapid return to prior levels of fitness.
- Functional overreaching refers to a training stress that induces persistent fatigue that resolves after a few days of rest or reduced training load. Periodic functional overreaching is essential to promote the greatest gains in fitness.
- Nonfunctional overreaching occurs when the training load remains too high for too long, requiring a few weeks of rest or reduced training for performance to return to normal.
- Overtraining syndrome is the result of months of hard training (and other life stressors) that combine to create a prolonged state of mental and physical fatigue that can take many months of rest to resolve.
- Optimal adaptations and improvements in performance occur when the stimulus of training facilitated by rest, sleep, nutrition, and hydration produces cellular and systemic changes that improve the capacity for hard physical activity.

Review Questions

1. Identify and briefly describe the five principles of training program design.
2. Explain why periodic functional overreaching is important for maximizing the adaptations to training.
3. Describe the basic concepts involved with block periodization training.
4. Explain the concept of tapering before important competitions.
5. List three symptoms of overtraining and describe how overtraining differs from nonfunctional overreaching.

CHAPTER SIX

Training to Improve Strength and Muscle Mass

Objectives:

- Learn the ways in which muscles respond and adapt to strength training.
- Discover how nutrition influences responses to strength training.
- Understand how muscles respond to training, detraining, and retraining.

In this photo, you can see the bulging biceps muscles straining against the resistance of the barbell, with the forearm muscles also engaged to lock the wrist in place. Nerve impulses from the brain have activated motor units in the arm flexor muscles and in a variety of muscles in the torso and legs for stabilization. The man in the photo could likely complete many repetitions with this weight before fatiguing. If his goal is to build biceps strength and mass, how many sets and reps should he complete in a training session? How much weight should he lift? How many sessions each week? With strength training, when is the point of diminishing return? In other words, is strength training for an hour five times each week any better at building strength and mass than training for just two shorter sessions each week?

Techniques for increasing muscle strength have been a central part of sport training for centuries, so you'd think that by this time sport scientists and fitness trainers would have a clear idea of what works best for building strength and mass. They don't. In fact, there is healthy ongoing debate about how much and how often people should engage in strength training to optimize the cellular adaptations that lead to increased strength and muscle mass. That debate is fueled by inconsistent research findings. To begin this chapter, let's revisit the adaptations that are needed for increased strength and mass.

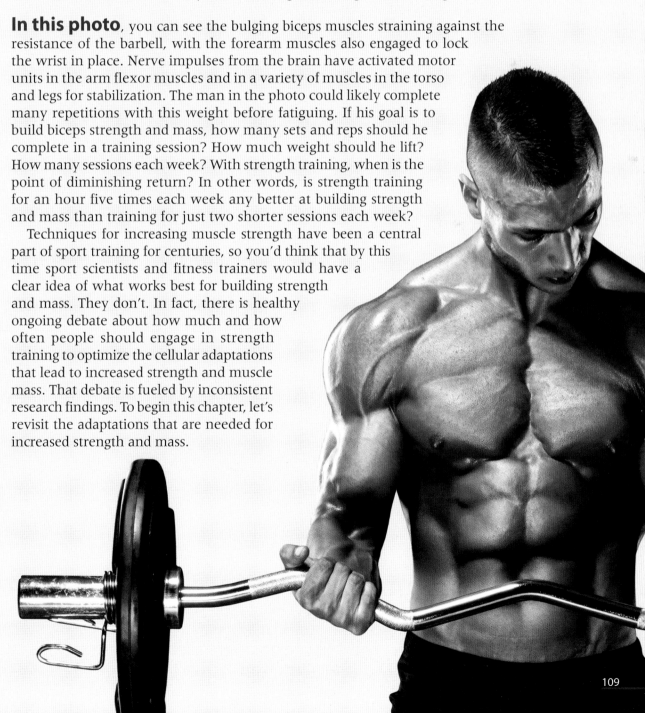

How Do Strength and Mass Increase?

As you remember from chapter 1, several adaptations to strength training occur in the central nervous system and in muscle cells.

In people who are new to strength training or haven't engaged in strength training for a few months or longer, muscle strength increases soon after training begins. That increase in strength has nothing to do with an increase in contractile proteins and everything to do with increased recruitment of motor units. In other words, muscle strength is not all about muscle size. As the nervous system recruits more motor units, force production (strength) increases because more muscle cells are involved in each contraction. After the first 8 to 10 weeks, muscle cells adapt to the continuing stress of strength training by creating more proteins (actin, myosin, troponin, tropomyosin, titin, and many others), and muscle mass increases. How much muscle mass and strength are added as a result of strength training depends on the factors shown in figure 6.1.

The most important influence on the amount of muscle mass that results from strength training is genetics. It's obvious that some people have the genetic predisposition to add large amounts of muscle mass, whereas others do not. The extent to which a person can add muscle mass is primarily determined by genotype (inherited genetic makeup), which establishes an upper limit of sorts for muscle mass and all other characteristics of cells, a good example of how nature determines what nurture (strength training, in this case) can accomplish. However, everyone can add at least some mass and increase muscle strength with the proper training program. That's because phenotype is determined by the interaction of genotype and environment. In the case of muscle mass, environment includes factors such as the extent of physical activity in childhood, age of starting strength training, duration of strength training, diet, and current methods of strength training. Age and sex also play roles.

Training of any sort alters phenotype, at least until training ceases and the adaptations gradually disappear. The stimulus of strength training is intended to provoke an adaptive response: The addition of functional proteins to muscle cells, which enables greater force production as

well as an increase in the size of individual cells and consequently the entire muscle. Strength training triggers signals within the muscle cell that stimulate the cell nuclei to churn out more contractile proteins that are then added in parallel to the existing contractile proteins in the cell. In other words, effective strength training causes an increase in muscle protein synthesis. Training increases the interaction of the muscle cell's signaling pathways with the DNA residing in the many nuclei within each muscle cell. Genotype determines how responsive muscle nuclei will be to training and therefore how many new muscle proteins will be added before reaching the upper limit imposed by your genotype.

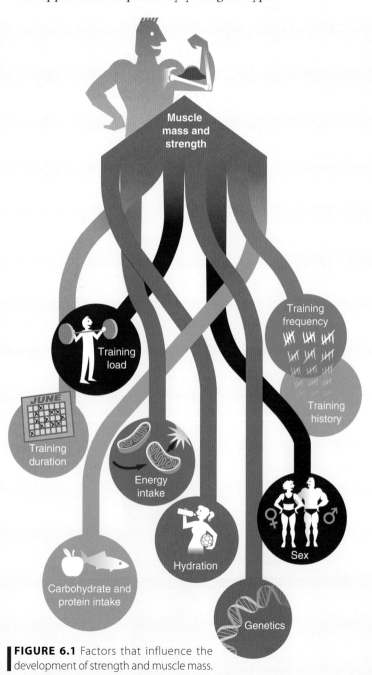

FIGURE 6.1 Factors that influence the development of strength and muscle mass.

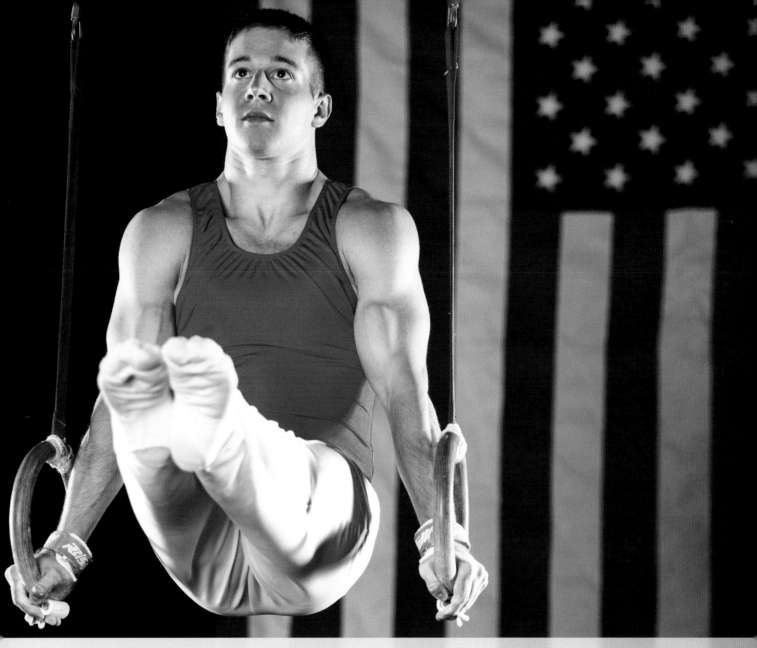

Adaptations to Strength Training

- More motor units recruited
- Greater stimulation frequency of motor units
- More synchronous recruiting of motor units
- Reduced inhibition of motor units
- Increased size of muscle cells (hypertrophy)
- Possibly a small increase in number of muscle cells (hyperplasia)
- Improved mitochondrial function
- Increased capillarization
- Increased bone mineral density and bone strength
- Increased strength of ligaments and tendons

Causes of Muscle Hypertrophy

- More contractile proteins (actin and myosin)
- More structural proteins
- More elastic proteins
- More sarcoplasm
- More myofibril units
- More connective tissue
- More intracellular water (75%-80% of muscle mass is water)
- More muscle cells (possible but not usual)

Examples of Options for Strength Training

- Body weight exercises
- Strength training machines (many different options)
- Free weights (barbells and dumbbells)
- Body bars
- Kettlebells
- Elastic bands
- Weighted balls
- Weighted clubs
- Eccentric, concentric, and isometric exercises
- Ballistic movements
- Unilateral and bilateral exercises
- Strength training straps

Can Women Increase Strength Without Dramatically Increasing Muscle Mass?

The simple answer is yes. Remember that significant gains in muscle strength occur early in training before muscle mass has a chance to increase. Those strength gains are associated with the recruitment of more motor units and other changes within the nervous system. Women who want to gain strength and improve muscle function but do not want to develop large muscles can train with lighter weights and tailor their long-term training program accordingly. In brief, the extent of the increase in muscle size is determined by genetics and the type of strength training. Another important factor in determining how much muscle mass is added as a result of training is testosterone production. Testosterone is an anabolic and androgenic steroid hormone. In other words, testosterone promotes anabolic responses such as the gain in mass and strength that accompanies resistance training as well as androgenic responses such as the growth of body hair and lower voice that accompany puberty in boys.

Estrogen, the primary sex hormone in females, is produced directly from testosterone. For that reason, all females produce testosterone in small quantities (20 times less than men produce). As a result, the anabolic responses to strength training in women are muted compared to the responses in men, who benefit from higher testosterone levels. Estrogen is produced in the ovaries and fat cells from testosterone, which is produced from cholesterol. The impact of estrogen on muscles and connective tissues in response to training is not well understood.

The table of various programs shows how strength training workouts can be customized to match the goals of the athlete or client. These examples illustrate how training can be modified to meet individuals' interests and goals.

Level	Goal	Upper-body muscles	Lower-body muscles
16-year-old female swimmer	Increase strength to swim faster Lose excess fat weight	Lat pull-down machine Assisted pull-ups Single-arm cable pull-downs	Kettlebell squats Weighted hip thrusts Hamstring curls Box jumps
		Following early season instruction on proper technique and two weeks of reps with light weight, transition to 3 sets of 3-15 reps with progressively heavier weights over time.	
22-year-old female beginner	Transition from sedentary to active lifestyle Improve muscle tone Lose excess fat weight	Lat pull-down machine Seated row machine Reverse fly with light tension band	Leg press Body-weight step-up Leg extension
		3 sets of 15-20 reps Moderate weight with 60-90 sec rest	
32-year-old female fitness enthusiast	Increase muscle strength. Increase muscle definition without adding too much lean mass Increase stamina for fitness classes	Assisted chin-up Dumbbell row Cable crossover reverse fly	Barbell back squat Weighted reverse lunge Lunge jump
		3 sets of 12-15 reps Moderate to heavy weight with 30-45 sec rest	
52-year-old female competitive tri-athlete	Increase strength for triathlon performance Willing to gain some lean mass	Assisted chin-up* Dumbbell prone lying pullover Single-arm low cable row with rotation	Barbell front squat Weighted step-up with reverse lunge Med-ball squat jump
		3 sets of 3-15 reps Moderate to heavy weight with 90-120 sec rest *Work to failure, then perform 3 successive negative reps	

Workouts were created by Kelly Schnell, BS, CSCS, ACSM-CPT, Inspyr Fitness, Arlington Heights, IL.

What's the Best Way to Gain Strength and Mass?

Muscles are very plastic. No, muscles aren't *made* of plastic, but muscles do have a remarkable ability to adapt very quickly to varying conditions, a feature known as *plasticity*. Muscles start slowly adapting within hours of training and, on the other end of the spectrum, begin to slowly lose those adaptations within hours of no training. When a limb is put in a cast or when a person is confined to bed for long periods, muscle cells atrophy—that is, they experience almost an immediate loss of contractile proteins and lose size and strength, a loss that can amount to 3% to 4% each day.

You have already learned that muscle cells increase their content of functional proteins in response to training, an adaptation that allows the cells to increase their capacity for doing work. This increase in functional protein content continues for as long as the muscles are progressively overloaded, eventually plateauing at a limit set by genotype. Too much strength training too soon not only increases the risk of injury but also leads to overreaching and perhaps overtraining, conditions discussed in chapter 5. Just the right amount of training leads to gradual but progressive increases in strength and mass. So what is just the right amount of strength training? How many sets? How many reps? How often?

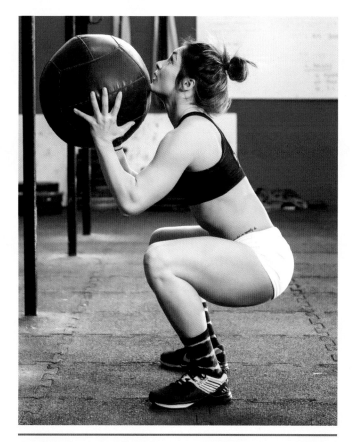

Strength training exposes muscles to a variety of stimuli that interact to produce an increase in muscle protein synthesis. Those stimuli include mechanical stress on muscle cells; increased motor unit recruitment; swelling of active muscle cells; the influence of hormones such as testosterone, growth hormone, and insulin-like growth factor (IGF-1); minor damage to muscle cells; the accumulation of metabolites such as lactic acid; and the increased production of free radicals (e.g., reactive oxygen species). All these stimuli interact to determine the overall increase in muscle protein synthesis.

General Guidelines for Resistance Training Programs

Based on the available research, here are some practical tips around which strength training programs should be designed. These concepts and suggestions apply regardless of the goal of the strength training program, be it for someone starting a fitness program, an athlete seeking to improve sport-specific strength, or a bodybuilder striving to add muscle mass. Of course, an important caveat is that everyone should first learn proper exercise technique. Those new to resistance training should first opt for strength exercises that develop basic resistance training skills before moving on to more sophisticated techniques. Endless variations in strength training programs can be developed around these principles, so these tips should be considered the building blocks for designing and individualizing strength training.

■ *Everyone is different.* Your genes determine how much and how quickly strength and mass will develop. Even if the training load is the same, athletes will experience different rates and amounts of improvement.

■ *Keep it simple.* Complicated, periodized, movement-specific regimens are no better at building strength and mass than are simpler, yet challenging, approaches.

■ *Twice per week is effective.* This is particularly true for intense sessions that demand exhaustive efforts. That does not mean that athletes can't or shouldn't strength train more frequently if they choose. It does mean that exhaustive training of individual muscle groups more than twice each week will not produce dramatically greater gains in strength and mass. In other words, a strength training program that works the arms, shoulders, chest, and back on Mondays and Wednesdays, and the abdominals, gluteals, and legs on Tuesdays and Thursdays, effectively works those muscle groups two days per week.

■ *At least one set, 3 to 15 reps.* Lifting a weight heavy enough to cause muscles to tire after just 3 to 15 repetitions also provides a strong stimulus that will increase strength and mass. Of course, heavy resistance isn't for everyone, so if multiple sets with more than 15 reps are needed, that too will lead to gains in strength and mass, provided that the muscle groups are stressed frequently enough. For example, a strength training program for a football lineman might include 3 sets of 8 reps with heavy resistance, while a defensive back on the same team might complete a warm-up and then 1 or 2 sets of 20 reps with lighter resistance but faster contractions. See table 6.1 later in this chapter for one example of a 20-minute strength training workout for increasing strength and mass.

■ *Strive to fail.* Regardless of how many sets and reps you choose to do, periodically achieving momentary *muscle failure* helps stimulate strength gains. Working to momentary failure—whether with 3 reps or 30 reps—increases the number of motor units recruited, ensuring an adequate stimulus for adaptations to occur.

■ *Stay steady.* Keep all movements smooth and steady in both directions to maximally stress the muscles. Doing so increases the muscles' *time under tension*, helping ensure an adequate training stimulus. Lifting too rapidly creates momentum that reduces the overall stimulative stress on the muscle and yet increases the risk of injury. Athletes should rest enough between sets to ensure consistent form.

▌ *Enjoy the challenge.* Choose a type of resistance training that keeps you coming back for more. Feel free to change to another approach when you get bored and begin to slack off in your training.

▌ *Equipment doesn't matter.* Use whatever equipment is available. There is no doubt that some types of exercise equipment have advantages in terms of comfort, stability, range of motion, joint forces, equipment footprint, and other factors, but fancy equipment is not needed for building strength. If you doubt that, arm-wrestle a farmer sometime.

▌ *One limb at a time can help.* Whether it's a chest press, a biceps curl, or a squat, training only one arm or leg at a time (*unilateral training*) requires engagement of the core muscles for stabilization. That means multiple muscle groups get a workout, and that is a good thing for overall strength development.

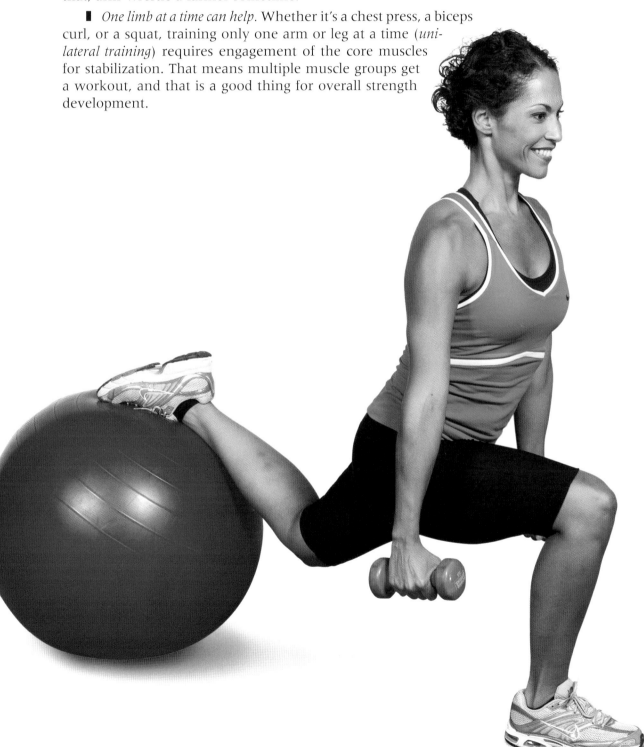

■ *For strength and power gains.* Use high loads or resistance (e.g., >80% 1RM) with fewer reps and sets (e.g., 3 sets of 8 reps). 1RM is the maximal load or resistance an athlete can accomplish in one effort.

■ *For size/mass gains.* Emphasize multiple (3 or more) sessions per week. Rely on more repetitions (e.g., 3 sets of 25 reps) and work to momentary muscle failure. Sessions can include both low loads and high loads to add variety.

■ *Take some rest.* Between hard sets, rest for a minute or two to allow muscles time to recuperate before the next hard effort. Remember, it is important to recruit as many motor units as possible and sufficient rest between sets helps achieve that.

■ *Mix it up.* There is no need to repeat the same exercises for months on end. As long as muscles are adequately stressed, increases in strength and mass will occur. In fact, no one type of strength training is sufficient to meet all the strength-related demands of sport and physical activity. For that reason, it makes scientific sense to expose athletes to a variety of different resistance training exercises.

■ *Your parents are the ones to blame (or thank).* Your genotype determines how you respond to exercise, and strength training is no exception. Those who quickly become stronger and more toned have their parents to thank. Those who work harder than everyone else and see only a fraction of the improvement have their parents to blame.

■ *Embrace muscle soreness; avoid muscle pain.* Periodic soreness will occur whenever the training load is increased or new exercises are introduced. That kind of soreness is a normal response. Pain in muscles and joints that limits movements is not normal.

■ *No one way is best.* Athletes can develop muscle strength, mass, leanness, and tone in a number of different ways. For example, construction workers, farmers, and other laborers develop impressive functional strength not by adhering to the conventional principles of resistance training but by stressing their muscles with varied loads on a daily basis. Their muscles regularly tire, burn, ache, experience soreness, and gradually adapt to the stress of the job. The moral to this story is that muscles taken out of their comfort zone on a regular basis respond with increased strength and mass.

■ *Protein is your friend.* Water and carbohydrate are your friends, too. A hydrated muscle is an anabolic muscle, so staying hydrated throughout the day promotes muscle anabolism. After a workout, tired muscles need carbohydrate to replenish their energy stores and protein to jump-start muscle repair and growth. Normal meals and snacks provide those nutrients, but consuming a large glass of chocolate milk or similar protein drink immediately after a workout will quickly supply muscles with the protein and carbohydrate needed for recovery and growth. Optimizing muscle protein synthesis is not just for power lifters and bodybuilders. Optimizing protein synthesis simply means to create the ideal environment for muscle recovery, repair, and adaptation.

Resources for Information on Strength Training Science

- American College of Sports Medicine (ACSM; www.acsm.org)
- American Council on Exercise (ACE; www.acefitness.org)
- Collegiate Strength and Conditioning Coaches association (CSCCa; www.cscca.org)
- IDEA Health and Fitness Association (IDEA; www.ideafit.com)
- National Athletic Trainers Association (www.nata.org)
- National Strength and Conditioning Association (NSCA; www.nsca.com)

Performance Nutrition Spotlight

Research has shown that consuming just 20-40 grams (80-160 kcal) of high-quality protein (dairy, lean meat, fish, eggs, soy) soon after a hard workout is enough to maximally stimulate muscle protein synthesis.

If maximum strength and muscle mass were the most important determinants of athletic success, power lifters and bodybuilders would dominate all sports. Athletes benefit by improving functional strength so they can apply greater muscle force, power, and endurance when and where it matters most to performance in their sports. Athletes can gain strength—and often at least a little muscle mass—through normal training in their sports. Further increasing strength through resistance training can boost performance if the gain in strength augments the forces required for success in that sport. That does not mean that resistance training has to mimic the exact movements in sports. It does mean that, for instance, if triceps strength is an important component of a sport movement, then increasing triceps strength through a variety of resistance exercises is likely to contribute to improved performance. In addition, people who strength-train will reap benefits over and above improved sports performance.

Time crunch? Table 6.1 is a sample program based on the previous strength training concepts that provides an effective full-body workout in just 20 minutes. The only equipment needed is a set of dumbbells. In this workout, transition immediately from one exercise to the next, and increase the resistance once you achieve 15 reps in the max set. Emphasize proper form and use a spotter when needed.

> The highest rate of muscle growth in response to strength training is about a 1% per week increase in muscle mass.

Performance Nutrition Spotlight

Tart cherry juice, beet juice, and pomegranate juice all have antioxidant and anti-inflammatory properties that can reduce exercise-induced muscle damage (EIMD) and DOMS. For example, consuming 8 ounces (237 ml) of tart cherry juice twice a day has been shown to reduce muscle pain and markers of inflammation, while speeding the return of strength after EIMD. Consuming omega-3 fatty acids has also been reported to promote recovery from EIMD.

Benefits of Strength Training

- Better joint stabilization
- Improved balance
- Lower risk of falls
- Increased resting metabolic rate (RMR)
- Improved physical appearance
- Increased bone mineral density
- Reduced risk of osteoporosis
- Improved blood lipid profile
- Faster recovery from injury, illness, and surgery
- Better sleep
- Improved cardiovascular health
- Reduced risk of depression
- Stronger self-esteem
- Improved glucose metabolism
- Reduced blood pressure
- Better insulin sensitivity

TABLE 6.1   **20-Minute Whole-Body Workout for Strength and Mass**

Exercise	Warm-up set	Max set
Right-arm curl	1 set of 10 reps, light weight	1 set of 3-15 reps, heavy weight
Left-arm row	1 set of 10 reps, light weight	1 set of 3-15 reps, heavy weight
Abs (plank, crunch)	30 sec	30 sec
Right-arm triceps kickback	1 set of 10 reps, light weight	1 set of 3-15 reps, heavy weight
Left-arm chest press	1 set of 10 reps, light weight	1 set of 3-15 reps, heavy weight
Abs (plank, crunch)	30 sec	30 sec
Left-leg squat	1 set of 10 reps, light weight	1 set of 3-15 reps, heavy weight
Right-arm chest press	1 set of 10 reps, light weight	1 set of 3-15 reps, heavy weight
Abs (plank, crunch)	30 sec	30 sec
Left-arm triceps kickback	1 set of 10 reps, light weight	1 set of 3-15 reps, heavy weight
Right-arm row	1 set of 10 reps, light weight	1 set of 3-15 reps, heavy weight
Abs (plank, crunch)	30 sec	30 sec
Left-arm curl	1 set of 10 reps, light weight	1 set of 3-15 reps, heavy weight
Right-leg squat	1 set of 10 reps, light weight	1 set of 3-15 reps, heavy weight

How Do Anabolic Hormones Work?

Anabolic hormones include testosterone, growth hormone, insulin, and insulin-like growth factor-1 (IGF-1), all of which can turn on protein synthesis in muscle cells. The concentration of anabolic hormones in the bloodstream naturally increases soon after a training session (and at other times in the day), although that response is not needed to increase strength and mass. However, it didn't take unscrupulous athletes, coaches, scientists, and physicians long to figure out that the natural limits imposed by genotype could be exceeded with pharmacology. Most anabolic steroids that athletes use to illicitly improve performance are substances that mimic the effects of testosterone. In addition to the natural precursors of testosterone such as DHEA and androstenedione, numerous designer steroids are produced by making small alterations to the structure of the testosterone molecule. Other anabolic molecules such as insulin, growth hormone (GH), and insulin-like growth factor 1 (IGF-1) are essential hormones that support many normal bodily functions by stimulating the nuclei in cells to produce proteins such as enzymes, signaling molecules, structural proteins, and contractile proteins. When muscle cells are exposed to higher-than-normal levels of anabolic hormones, peptides, and growth factors, the cell nuclei produce more proteins, adding to the protein-producing stimulus created by strength training.

Using anabolic steroids (testosterone and its natural precursors or synthetic analogs) to augment performance is clearly cheating because such doping creates an unfair competitive advantage. In addition, using anabolic steroids is associated with a variety of health risks that include liver damage, enlarged prostate gland, reduced stature (among young athletes), testicular atrophy, reduced sperm count, enlarged male breasts (termed *gynecomastia*), acne, masculinization of females, disrupted menstruation, growth of facial hair, breast atrophy, psychological issues, and deepening of the voice. Long-term use of growth hormone is associated with cardiomyopathy, acromegaly (enlarged skull), hypertension, heart disease, and weakening of joints and connective tissues. These negative consequences should not be surprising, because interfering with the intricate control of hormonal function by indiscriminate doping is bound to disrupt normal cellular function.

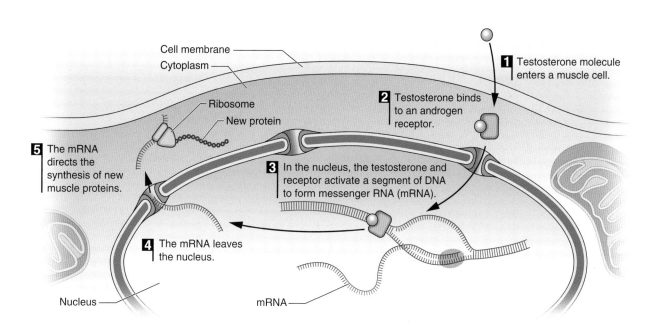

Steroids stimulate muscle cell nuclei to produce more contractile proteins, adding to the stimulus created by strength training.

How Important Is the Type of Muscle Contraction?

When it comes to strength training, variety is a good thing. It's psychologically refreshing to be faced with a new challenge periodically, along with different equipment and exercise variation to stress muscles in varied ways. Free weights, machine weights, elastic bands, stability balls, kettlebells, weighted balls, and other equipment all have a legitimate place in a strength training program (see figure 6.2).

It is important to remember that muscle cells can contract in various ways that affect overall motor unit recruitment and force production. For example, the concentric contractions needed to lift a weight require that muscle cells shorten, with actin and myosin filaments sliding over one another, creating a bulging muscle with each repetition. When that weight is slowly lowered, the muscle cells lengthen (eccentric contraction) while still producing force as the actin and myosin filaments continue to interact and the elastic connective tissue and tendons of the muscle are stretched, contributing to force production. In isometric contractions, the joint is held in a fixed position while muscle cells shorten and then maintain a sustained contraction. Most sports require a dynamic, ever-changing combination of all three types of contractions, and strength training programs should include exercises that mimic those conditions. The use of unstable surfaces such as balance boards and vibration platforms adds more psychological challenge and physical stress to exercise. This challenge may augment strength development and adds interest and variety to a training program.

FIGURE 6.2 Various types of equipment and muscle contractions create variety and stress muscles in different ways.

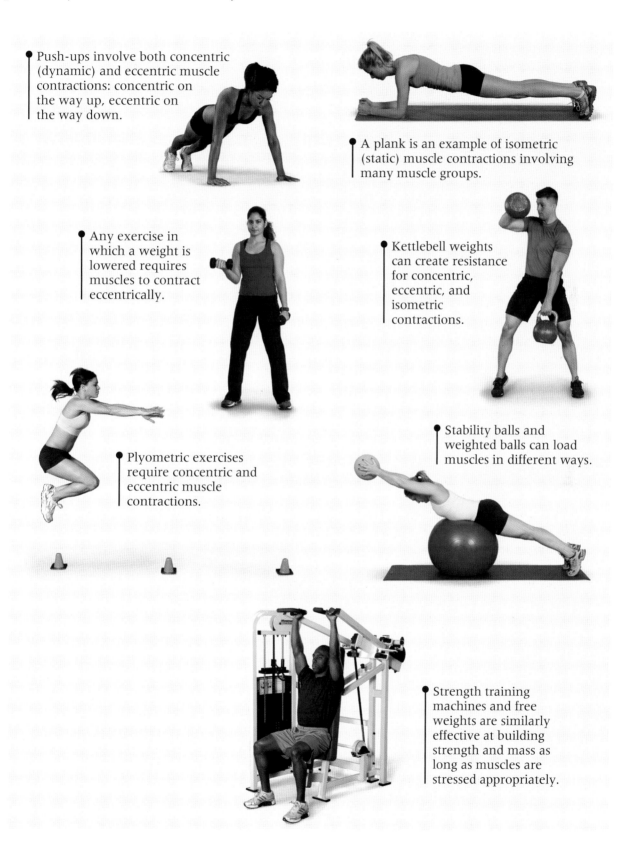

Push-ups involve both concentric (dynamic) and eccentric muscle contractions: concentric on the way up, eccentric on the way down.

A plank is an example of isometric (static) muscle contractions involving many muscle groups.

Any exercise in which a weight is lowered requires muscles to contract eccentrically.

Kettlebell weights can create resistance for concentric, eccentric, and isometric contractions.

Plyometric exercises require concentric and eccentric muscle contractions.

Stability balls and weighted balls can load muscles in different ways.

Strength training machines and free weights are similarly effective at building strength and mass as long as muscles are stressed appropriately.

Eccentric training is not only for athletes and weightlifters. Because eccentric contractions require less energy and result in less cardiovascular discomfort, they are well suited in programs for those who are rehabilitating from injury, for older adults, and for those suffering from health and neuromuscular issues (see table 6.2). The delayed-onset muscle soreness (DOMS) that often occurs with eccentric training can be avoided or lessened by slowly increasing the eccentric workload over time (a good example of the principle of progressive overload). One challenge with eccentric strength training is to expose muscles to enough resistance to optimally stimulate the muscle. For example, curling a heavy weight (concentric contraction) places a lot of stress on the biceps but lowering that same weight (eccentric contraction) is much less of a stress. Fewer motor units and therefore fewer muscle cells are activated during lowering; some of the force produced is due to flexing of the myosin heads and the stretching of titin and other elastic molecules. Interestingly, eccentric training stimulates different signaling pathways inside muscle cells and results in different gene expression compared to concentric training. If the load in eccentric training is equal to that in concentric training, improvements in muscle strength and size are similar, if not slightly greater. Some specialized strength training equipment is designed to apply greater force during the eccentric phases of exercise so that there is an equal activation of motor units compared to the concentric phase, thereby increasing the overall training stimulus.

One response to strength training is an increase in the production of prostaglandins, molecules that influence the overall adaptation to training. The primary enzyme responsible for prostaglandin production is cyclooxygenase (COX). COX activity is inhibited by nonsteroidal anti-inflammatory drugs (NSAIDs) such as naproxen, ibuprofen, and aspirin, leading to the concern that consuming NSAIDs on a regular basis—as some athletes do—might reduce the benefits of strength training by blunting part of the adaptation response. Fortunately, research indicates that NSAID use at normal doses does not seem to negatively influence the development of muscle strength and mass.

TABLE 6.2 **Benefits and Risks of Eccentric Strength Training**

Benefits	Risks
Greater force production	Greater exercise-induced muscle damage
Increased anabolic signaling	Greater delayed-onset muscle soreness (DOMS; myalgia)
Lower energy cost	Temporary decrease in strength after a training session
More satellite cell activity	Reduced joint range of motion due to muscle swelling
Less cardiovascular stress and discomfort	Temporarily disrupted movement patterns
Lower perceived exertion	Temporarily impaired performance
Less fatigue	Increased risk of injury to muscles, joints, and bones
More motor cortex involvement	
Increased motor-unit recruitment	
Rapid gains in strength and mass	
Increased resting metabolic rate	
Improved blood lipid profile	
Better insulin sensitivity	

Based on S. Hody et al. "Eccentric Muscle Contractions: Risks and Benefits," *Frontiers in Physiology* 10, no. 536 (2019): 1-18.

Performance Nutrition Spotlight

Strength training in the evening followed by consuming 20 grams of high-quality protein will increase muscle protein synthesis during sleep more than consuming the protein in the absence of strength training.

Everyone involved in strength training would like to find a competitive edge—a quicker way to develop strength and mass. Endless ads in magazines and online tout shortcuts to superior strength with claims not necessarily based on superior science. Here are three examples:

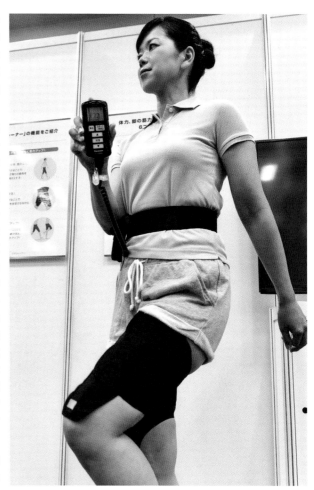

1. Electrical stimulation. The idea behind this technique is that if muscles can be stimulated to contract through electrodes placed on the skin, using an electrode device could augment or replace strength training. Electrical stimulation is widely used in patients whose limbs are immobilized by casts after injury or surgery with the purpose of reducing the loss of strength and mass. However, there is no good evidence that electrical stimulation of muscles will increase strength or mass, because the stimulation generally produces submaximal contractions, an inadequate stimulus compared to a well-designed strength training routine. In theory, if electrical stimulation were used to produce a supramaximal contraction during strength training, it might induce greater gains in strength and mass. That sounds good in theory, but the practical downside is that the pain, muscle damage, and potential for injury associated with supramaximal electrical stimulation far outweigh the benefits.

2. Restricted blood flow. Another way to increase the stimulus to muscles during strength training is to use occlusion training, which restricts blood flow to the muscles with just enough pressure to reduce venous blood flow so that muscle metabolites temporarily accumulate. For those who cannot lift heavy weights (a load of at least 80% of 1RM) because of age, illness, or injury, using a pressure cuff to reduce blood flow while lifting light weights (e.g., just 30% of 1RM) can theoretically increase the stimulus and produce greater gains in strength and mass. Reducing the blood flow to muscles during strength training may also stimulate the recruitment of motor units that are not usually involved in training, thereby enhancing the training effect. In fact, research indicates that occlusion training with light weights does result in increased strength and mass, a real benefit for those who are limited in their ability to lift heavier weights. Restricting blood flow in healthy individuals might provide some variety in training, but the real benefit appears to be for people who are restrained in one way or another in their ability to participate in conventional strength training.

3. Compression clothing. Clothing designed to compress muscle groups such as the thigh and calf muscles has been developed to aid muscle function in training and competition. The premise is that the right amount of compression can improve blood flow through the muscles, stabilize muscle groups, and perhaps add an element of elasticity to augment jumping, sprinting, and other explosive movements. Research on sport compression clothing has produced mixed results, with most studies reporting no benefits to performance or recovery. However, no one has ever been harmed by sport compression clothing, so if the garment feels good to wear, that alone might be enough of a benefit to justify the cost of the clothing.

What's the Role of Nutrition?

Those interested in increasing strength and mass are often interested in how nutrition—especially protein nutrition—can help. This is an interesting area of sport science, and the research is clear that consuming high-quality protein after a workout will optimize muscle protein synthesis. From a practical perspective, that means consuming protein soon after a workout. The body digests protein into a variety of amino acids that are absorbed into the bloodstream. High-quality protein contains all the essential amino acids—most important the amino acid leucine and others the body cannot make—that muscles need to increase the synthesis of proteins such as the contractile, structural, transport, and regulatory proteins required for increased strength and mass. During workouts, muscle protein breakdown increases, a natural response to exercise. After workouts, it makes sense to consume protein to increase protein synthesis to help speed muscle recovery, repair, and adaptation. Doing so on a regular basis accelerates increases in strength and mass. It also makes sense to consume protein snacks periodically during the day to bump up protein synthesis to further support the production of functional proteins in muscle.

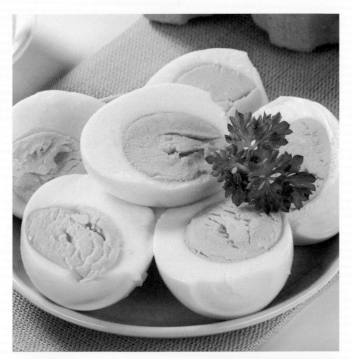

Research demonstrates that 20 grams of high-quality protein found in milk, meat, eggs, and fish seems sufficient to maximally stimulate muscle protein synthesis after exercise. Older people (i.e., >50 years) demonstrate what researchers have termed *anabolic resistance* to protein intake in that they require 40 grams of protein for maximal stimulation of protein synthesis. The combination of exercise and protein intake is particularly important with aging because it helps protect against the loss of muscle mass, contributes to bone health, and aids in appetite control. A related benefit is that research shows that the stronger tend to live longer.

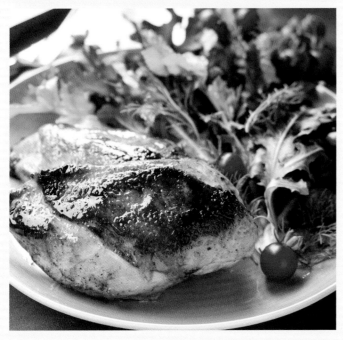

Food Servings That Contain 20 Grams of High-Quality Protein

- 3 eggs (240 kcal)
- 3 ounces (85 g) turkey (90 kcal)
- 3 ounces (85 g) canned tuna (85 kcal)
- 3 ounces (85 g) chicken (90 kcal)
- 4.5 ounces (125 g) ham (125 kcal)
- 3.5 ounces (105 g) lean beef (130 kcal)
- 6 ounces (180 g) cottage cheese (160 kcal)
- 4 ounces (115 g) ground beef (200 kcal)
- 2.6 ounces (76 g) seitan (110 kcal)

There is growing evidence that distributing protein intake evenly throughout the day, including before bedtime, will maximize muscle protein synthesis and help maintain or increase muscle mass. For example, if a 180-pound (82 kg) athlete consumes 180 grams of protein per day, that protein intake can be divided into four portions, each containing 45 grams of protein, as part of three regular meals and a snack before bedtime. Consuming protein in that manner has been shown to sustain higher rates of muscle protein synthesis. You should not worry about precisely spreading protein intake across the day; simply remember to consume some protein at each meal and snack.

Any time you complete a hard workout, there are surges in a variety of hormones in the bloodstream, part of the natural response to exercise. In addition, any time you eat a snack or meal, a hormonal response accompanies the ingestion of foods and beverages. Advertisements for some dietary supplements contain claims that the supplement provokes an increase in anabolic hormones that help increase strength and mass. If only it were that simple! Research shows that the hormonal response to resistance training and to the ingestion of dietary supplements does not play a critical role in developing strength and mass. There's no doubt that the hormonal response to exercise and diet is important, but many other factors that occur in the days, weeks, and months of a training program have a far greater effect in the development of strength and mass.

Interestingly, increases in circulating anabolic hormones after exercise are less important than the number of androgen receptors in the muscle cell for stimulating gains in strength and mass. Women have much lower circulating testosterone at rest, and following resistance exercise the increase in testosterone is 45 times less in women than that experienced by men. Yet even with less circulating testosterone, women are able to increase muscle protein synthesis, muscle mass, and muscle strength. The increase in anabolic hormones that occurs after a workout is simply not that important.

> The temporary muscle hypertrophy that occurs during strength training is caused by the accumulation of fluid in and around muscle cells. This short-term increase in muscle size is one of many signals that help improve muscle strength and mass.

Detraining and Retraining

Muscle detraining can occur as a result of injury, illness, or simply stopping training. Injury, immobilization, and especially prolonged bed rest cause rapid changes in muscle that begin within hours. Muscle protein synthesis decreases and muscle cells begin to atrophy as contractile proteins are broken down. Strength loss can average 3% to 4% each day, as muscles become smaller and the nervous system loses some of its adaptations. Fortunately, retraining stimulates muscle growth and a return in strength. However, fully recovering strength and mass takes longer than the time spent in the period of disuse. Maintaining strength during an offseason or whenever normal training is disrupted can be achieved by one to two sessions each week, provided that the training stimulus is great enough.

Chapter Summary

- It is possible to develop muscle strength without substantial changes in muscle mass.
- The initial improvements in muscle strength are due to the increased recruitment of motor units.
- Muscle hypertrophy (increased muscle mass) occurs as a result of muscle cells adding contractile and other cellular proteins.
- There is no one resistance training technique or piece of equipment that is best for the development of muscle strength.
- A variety of factors interact to produce gains in strength and mass. Those factors include mechanical stress, fatigue, motor unit recruitment, muscle damage, metabolite accumulation, hormonal response, and other factors unique to each individual.
- Exercising to momentary muscle failure is a helpful but not mandatory feature of strength training.
- Ample dietary protein intake (1.2 to 2.0 grams of protein per kilogram of body weight per day) helps support the muscle protein synthesis required for increased strength and mass.
- Concentric, eccentric, and isometric training all result in improved strength provided the training load is sufficient.
- Muscles begin to lose strength after a couple weeks of detraining, but retraining will restore strength and reduced training (e.g., 1 to 2 sessions per week) can maintain strength.

Review Questions

1. Describe the reason for the improvements in muscle strength that occur before increases in muscle mass.
2. Briefly explain how strength training results in muscle hypertrophy.
3. Discuss the role of anabolic hormones in increasing the production of contractile proteins.
4. Describe the differences between concentric and eccentric strength training.
5. Explain how dietary protein helps enhance the responses to strength training.

CHAPTER SEVEN

Training for Weight Loss

Objectives

- Understand why moving more and eating less is a great starting point for losing fat because it is based on the energy balance equation.
- Understand the factors that can complicate the energy balance equation.
- Learn the basic principles of energy balance.
- Discover the factors that determine resting metabolic rate and daily energy expenditure.

At any given time, it seems as though there are hundreds of diets of various sorts that are touted to promote rapid weight loss. Add to that confusing scenario the countless advertisements for dietary supplements that promise the same miraculous results and then layer on weekly news flashes about the latest scientific discoveries that promise to ignite the body's fat-burning machinery, and that's just a glimpse of the information overload awaiting anyone interested in losing weight. Fortunately, the principles of effective weight loss—losing excess body fat and keeping it off—are not as complicated as they might appear. Changes in body weight—either up or down—occur because of changes in *energy balance*.

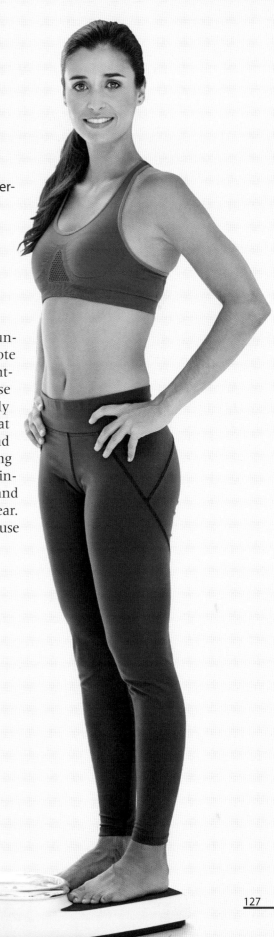

Weight Loss Is All About Energy Balance

You might recall from chapter 2 that the term energy refers to the capacity to do work. That work could be related to the contraction of a skeletal muscle cell, the transport of a glucose molecule across a membrane, the creation of an intracellular signal, or the synthesis of a functional protein such as an enzyme. All that work requires ATP, and ATP production requires the oxidation of glucose and fat.

Converting the energy in a glucose molecule or a fatty-acid molecule into ATP is inefficient; 50% of the energy in glucose and fat is lost as heat during the production of ATP. That inefficiency is not all bad, though, because that heat helps keep body temperature normal. (To keep things in perspective, the efficiency of the gasoline engine in a car is only 10% to 20%.)

The *first law of thermodynamics* indicates that energy is not created or destroyed; it simply changes from one form to another. As an example, the chemical energy in a glucose molecule is changed into the chemical energy in an ATP molecule that is changed into the mechanical energy of a muscle contraction that is changed into the kinetic energy of a body movement. No energy has been created or destroyed.

All the energy associated with human movement is due to the energy of the sun (review the beginning of chapter 2 if you need a quick refresher). The energy in the sun's radiation is transformed by plants into chemical energy (e.g., starch and sugar). We and other animals consume plants (and we also consume some of the animals) and thereby capture their chemical energy in the form of carbohydrate, fat, and protein.

The concept of energy balance is simple and irrefutable, yet maddeningly complicated in its application to weight loss, especially for those who are already very overweight or obese. For now, let's stick with the simple part. When energy intake (the food and drink you consume) is the same as energy output (your energy expenditure), the total amount of energy in your body remains unchanged (see figure 7.1). As a result, your body weight will remain unchanged (ignoring daily changes in body water).

● When energy intake is greater than energy output, the total energy content of the body increases, as does body weight.

● Just the opposite happens when energy intake is less than energy output: The total energy content of the body falls and so does weight.

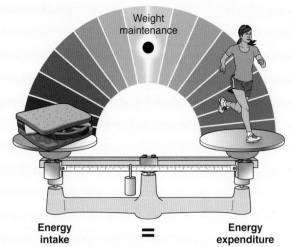

● The total energy content of the body is roughly the same as the total fat content of the body.

FIGURE 7.1 Energy balance is a simple concept that applies to everyone, yet not everyone responds in the same way to moving more and eating less.

Energy Input and Energy Output

On the energy intake (input) side of the equation, the key factor is the amount of energy you ingest as food and beverages. This energy is referred to as calories and is measured in Calories (kilocalories [kcal], which equals 1,000 calories). Energy intake actually means caloric intake, or how many calories you eat. Of course, many factors other than your energy expenditure (output) influence your energy balance, such as the availability of food, serving sizes, hunger and satiety hormones, and emotional connections with eating, to name a few.

On the energy output side of the equation, the number of calories you expend in a day is determined by an equally large number of factors. Fortunately, that large number can be reduced to four easy-to-understand categories: (1) resting metabolic rate, (2) thermic effect of food, (3) energy efficiency, and (4) physical activity energy expenditure. Figure 7.2 depicts those four components.

Overeating can lead to increased thermogenesis (heat production) because muscle and other cells increase fat oxidation and energy expenditure. Unfortunately, that thermogenesis cannot increase sufficiently to offset overeating. Simply put, the body is better at protecting against starvation than against gluttony.

❚ FIGURE 7.2 The four components of daily energy output.

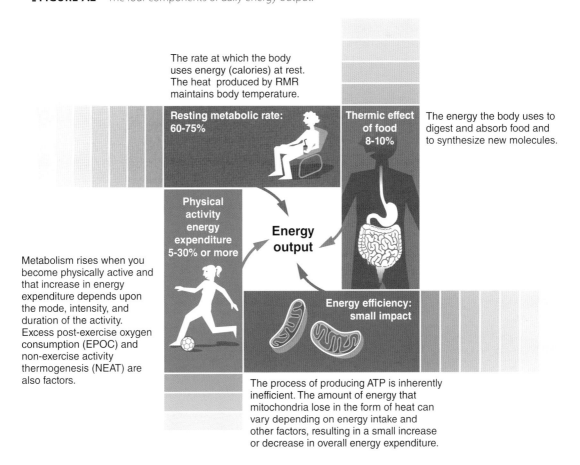

The rate at which the body uses energy (calories) at rest. The heat produced by RMR maintains body temperature.

Resting metabolic rate: 60-75%

Thermic effect of food 8-10%

The energy the body uses to digest and absorb food and to synthesize new molecules.

Physical activity energy expenditure 5-30% or more

Energy output

Energy efficiency: small impact

Metabolism rises when you become physically active and that increase in energy expenditure depends upon the mode, intensity, and duration of the activity. Excess post-exercise oxygen consumption (EPOC) and non-exercise activity thermogenesis (NEAT) are also factors.

The process of producing ATP is inherently inefficient. The amount of energy that mitochondria lose in the form of heat can vary depending on energy intake and other factors, resulting in a small increase or decrease in overall energy expenditure.

Resting metabolic rate (RMR) varies with body size and composition, and is affected by eating habits. RMR is influenced even by small movements, so fidgeting while sitting is enough to increase RMR. Most important, increasing muscle mass has a large impact on RMR because, as shown in figure 7.3, skeletal muscle accounts for at least 25% of RMR.

The *thermic effect of food* (TEF) refers to the energy used in digesting and absorbing food and beverages. TEF is affected by the size and composition of meals and the body's hormonal response to those meals, but only accounts for 8% to 10% of RMR.

Energy efficiency is another factor that influences daily energy expenditure. As noted at the beginning of this chapter, the ATP-producing processes in cells are not 100% efficient, because a lot of the energy associated with metabolism and muscle contraction is lost as heat. Producing more heat and less ATP is inefficient and that inefficiency increases fat and carbohydrate oxidation. That's bad for ATP production but good for weight loss.

One interesting factor involving energy efficiency is brown fat. Brown fat (brown adipose tissue) is commonly found in animals (especially hibernating animals such as bears). Brown fat cells have more mitochondria and capillaries compared to normal fat cells (white fat) and are inefficient in their production of ATP. The result is that brown fat cells break down a lot of fatty acids and produce a lot of heat, a handy advantage when you want to hibernate outdoors and you have enough body fat to last through the winter. Brown fat is also good for newborn babies. All humans are

> Resting metabolic rate is the amount of energy the body uses at rest and can be further broken down by the organ systems using the energy.

FIGURE 7.3 Resting metabolic rate (RMR) reflects the energy (calories) used by all body cells when the body is at rest.

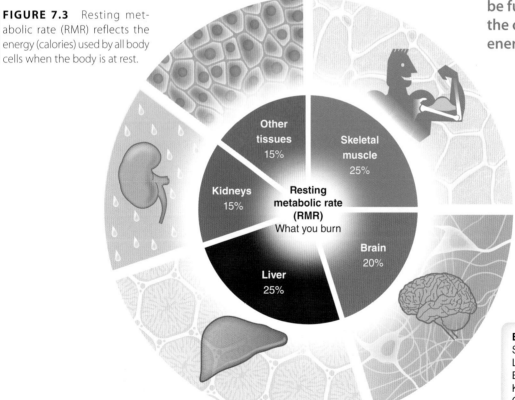

Resting metabolic rate (RMR)
What you burn

Other tissues 15%
Skeletal muscle 25%
Kidneys 15%
Brain 20%
Liver 25%

Example: RMR = 1600 kcal/day
Skeletal muscles use 400 kcal
Liver uses 400 kcal
Brain uses 320 kcal
Kidneys use 240 kcal
Other tissues use 240 kcal

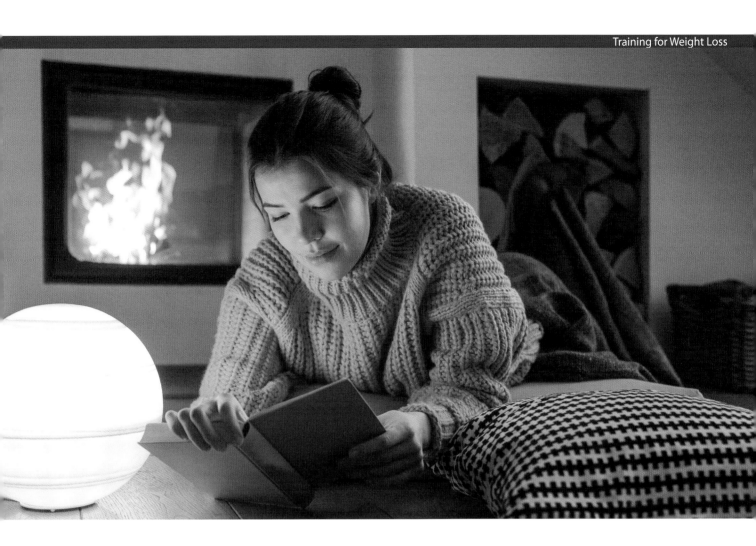

born with a small amount of brown fat (about 5% of body weight) to maintain body temperature after birth because infants can't fend for themselves in that regard. Brown fat is no longer needed as babies grow into toddlers because they are able to produce more heat by moving and they develop the capacity to shiver (a great way to produce heat).

However, adults do retain some brown fat. In fact, brown fat seems to increase in quantity as a result of prolonged exposure to cold weather. Beige fat cells appear to have characteristics between brown and white fat. This makes it theoretically possible that adults who have more brown or beige fat would have an easier time with weight control. You might have friends who seem to eat as much as they want and never gain weight. Could that be because they have more than their fair share of brown or beige fat? Having brown and beige fat may be one reason some people have an easier time losing or maintaining weight than others do. But, as in all things scientific, there are always additional reasons.

The topic of brown and beige fat is interesting not only for its potential connection to weight control but also because it is an example of how regular physical activity stimulates a variety of responses that influence tissues throughout the body. Skeletal muscles, heart muscles, and fat all release hormones and other proteins into the bloodstream during exercise, perhaps as a way to communicate their needs to other tissues. For example, during exercise, heart and skeletal muscles release a hormone called *irisin* that appears to promote the transformation of some white fat cells into beige fat cells. This is just one example of how active muscle can communicate with the brain, liver, kidneys, bone, pancreas, and fat cells to produce short- and long-term responses that benefit overall fitness and health.

Physical activity energy expenditure is a large factor within your control when it comes to weight management. The energy expended (calories burned) during physical activity depends on many factors such as the type of physical activity, intensity of the activity, duration of the activity, and body weight. Table 7.1 contains examples of how energy expenditure varies among activities. Notice that continuous activities that involve many muscles, such as running and swimming, usually have a higher energy cost than intermittent activities, such as tennis. Of course, someone who swims leisurely will expend fewer calories than someone playing an intense game of tennis, so the average values that you see in table 7.1 or find in other books or on the Internet are simply rough estimates of the average energy cost of activities.

Regular physical activity is the best single predictor of successful long-term weight loss.

TABLE 7.1 **Average Energy Cost of Physical Activities Expressed in Calories per Minute (kcal/min) and Relative to Body Weight (kcal/kg/min)**

Activity	Estimated kcal/min (derived from MET values, assuming 1 MET = 1.5 kcal/min)	Relative to body mass (kcal/kg/min)
Basketball game	12.0	0.123
Cycling		
Cycling hard uphill	21.0	0.071
Cycling flat terrain (<10.0 mph)	6.0	0.107
Cycling flat terrain (>20 mph)	24.0	0.343
Running		
12.1 km/h (7.5 mph)	14.0	0.200
16.1 km/h (10.0 mph)	18.0	0.260
Sitting	1.5	0.024
Sleeping	1.0	0.017
Standing	1.8	0.026
Swimming laps, freestyle, hard	15.0	0.285
Tennis, singles	12.0	0.101
Walking, 3.2 km/h (2.0 mph)	3.0	0.071
Resistance training, vigorous	9.0	0.117

Note: Values presented are for a 70-kilogram (154 lb) person. These values will vary depending on many other factors and should be viewed as estimates that can give athletes and clients a sense of how energy expenditure varies among activities. The energy cost of other activities can be found at https://sites.google.com/site/compendiumofphysicalactivities/ Activity-Categories.

Data from Ainsworth et al. Healthy Lifestyles Research Center, College of Nursing and Health Innovation, Arizona State University. https://sites.google.com/site/compendiumofphysicalactivities/Activity-Categories

Performance Nutrition Spotlight

For anyone interested in improving performance capacity, the American College of Sports Medicine recommends consuming 30 to 90 grams (120-360 kcal) of carbohydrate per hour during training and competition.

The estimates of energy cost displayed in online and in-store advertisements for exercise equipment such as treadmills, stationary bikes, and elliptical trainers are just that—estimates. Those values are based on a variety of equations that differ from one piece of equipment to another. For example, you might input your age and body weight into a treadmill to allow it to estimate your energy expenditure based on those two variables plus the treadmill speed and elevation. It is impossible to determine just how accurate those estimates are regarding your actual energy expenditure because the exercise equipment has no idea of how economically you are moving (reflected by your oxygen consumption at any given intensity), and you have no idea if the exercise equipment has been recently calibrated. So it's best to use that information only as general feedback.

Figure 7.4 depicts an interesting aspect of physical activity energy expenditure. *Nonexercise activity thermogenesis*, mercifully abbreviated as NEAT, can be thought of as accidental exercise because it encompasses the energy expended during daily activities such as standing, fidgeting, and stooping. You know people who just can't seem to sit still. Good for them, because fidgety people get a lot of accidental exercise; all those brief movements can add up to hundreds of calories each day.

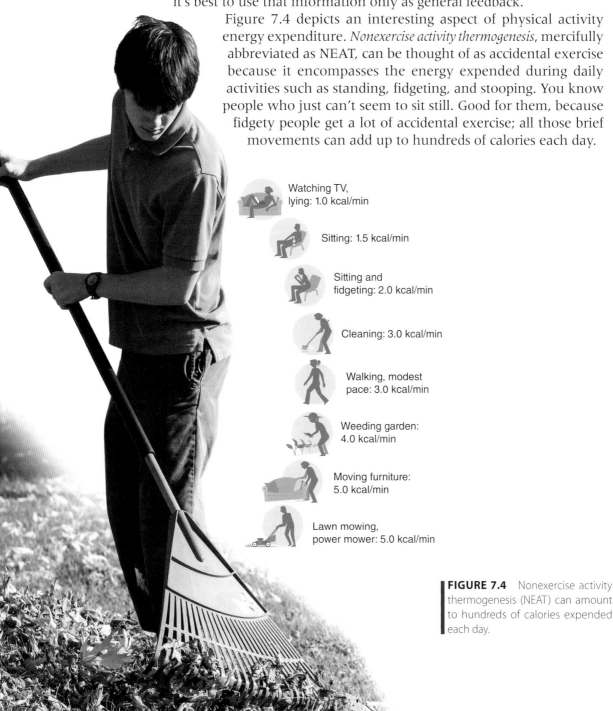

Watching TV, lying: 1.0 kcal/min

Sitting: 1.5 kcal/min

Sitting and fidgeting: 2.0 kcal/min

Cleaning: 3.0 kcal/min

Walking, modest pace: 3.0 kcal/min

Weeding garden: 4.0 kcal/min

Moving furniture: 5.0 kcal/min

Lawn mowing, power mower: 5.0 kcal/min

FIGURE 7.4 Nonexercise activity thermogenesis (NEAT) can amount to hundreds of calories expended each day.

What's the Best Way to Estimate RMR?

To help athletes and clients understand their daily energy (calorie) needs, it's helpful for them to understand their RMR. If you don't have access to equipment to measure oxygen consumption and lean body mass, then the next-best approach is to use equations to estimate RMR. Mobile phone apps and websites make the same estimates, so there's no need to belabor the topic here except to show that the equations look like those in table 7.2. To be most helpful, it makes sense to use more than one equation to create a range of RMR values that likely encompass the true RMR value for each person.

Measuring the resting metabolic rate (RMR) in a person who has severely restricted energy intake will underestimate true RMR because severe calorie restriction causes the metabolism in many tissues to slow down.

Weight-Loss Supplements

Hundreds of dietary supplements promise rapid weight loss. If that promise strikes you as too good to be true, that's because it is. Happily, this topic is a great example of the importance of the energy balance equation because the only way to lose fat weight is for energy intake to decrease or energy output to increase. For a dietary supplement to aid in fat loss would require the supplement to either reduce appetite (decrease energy intake) or increase resting metabolic rate (increase energy output). Is it possible for dietary supplements to do either? As you might imagine, a clear answer is hard to come by. Suffice it to say that the results of some studies of dietary supplements have shown small, short-lasting reductions in appetite and increases in resting metabolic rate that are not much different in magnitude from the results brought about by placebo. This is true of a variety of herbal preparations and ingredients such as forskolin and garcinia cambogia as well as green tea extract and other caffeine derivatives. The dietary supplements that do reduce appetite are those that contain prohibited or dangerous substances such as prescription drugs or designer stimulants. Weight-loss supplements have been found to contain sibutramine (an amphetamine analog now banned for use in humans), fluoxetine (Prozac, an anti-anxiety drug), phenolphthalein (a chemical reagent), triamterene (a prescription diuretic), and even sildenafil (Viagra). Supplement contamination with prescription drugs or banned substances is a widespread problem because it is next to impossible for most people to decipher ingredient labels or keep up with the news about weight-loss supplements. To help in that regard, the U.S. Food and Drug Administration issues e-mail alerts to interested consumers whenever a supplement tests positive for a prohibited substance (www.fda.gov/food/recalls-outbreaks-emergencies).

What's the Best Way to Estimate Daily Energy Needs?

The easiest way to estimate daily energy needs (caloric needs) is to multiply the estimate for RMR by a factor that roughly represents how active a person is on a daily basis. Again, it's most useful to a client or athlete to create a range of daily caloric needs based on a high- and low-activity estimate. Table 7.3 has an example using the volleyball player whose RMR was estimated in table 7.2. As with estimates of RMR, there are websites and phone apps that make similar calculations. Few people need the same amount of calories day after day because daily energy needs vary depending on activity. Note in table 7.3 that there is a 1,000-Calorie (kcal) difference in energy needs between the athlete's rest day and an intense training day.

TABLE 7.2 **Two Equations for Estimating RMR in Adults**

Equation	Men	Women	Example
Harris-Benedict	RMR (in kcal/day) = 66.473 + (13.7516 × body weight in kg) + (5.003 × height in cm) − (6.775 × age)	RMR (in kcal/day) = 665.0955 + (9.5634 × body weight in kg) + (1.8496 × height in cm) − (4.6756 × age)	20-year-old female volleyball player, 69 in. tall (175 cm), 136 lb (61.8 kg) RMR = 665.0955 + (9.5634 × 61.8) + (1.8496 × 175) − (4.6756 × 20) = 1,486 kcal/day
Mifflin-St. Jeor	RMR (in kcal/day) = (10 × body weight in kg) + (6.25 × height in cm) − (5 × age) + 5	RMR (in kcal/day) = (10 × body weight in kg) + (6.25 × height in cm) − (5 × age) − 161	20-year-old female volleyball player, 69 in. tall (175 cm), 136 lb (61.8 kg) RMR = (10 × 61.8) + (6.25 × 175) − (5 × 20) − 161 = 1,451 kcal/day

TABLE 7.3 **Estimating Daily Energy Needs From RMR and an Activity Factor**
Example: 20-year-old female volleyball player, 69 inches tall (175 cm), 136 pounds (61.8 kg)
Estimated average RMR = 1,469 kcal/day (the average of the two estimates in table 7.2)

Activity level	Activity factor	Energy needs
Rest day	RMR × 1.2	1,763 kcal
Light training day (e.g., ≤1 hr of light exercise)	RMR × 1.375	2,020 kcal
Moderate training day (e.g., 1 to 2 hr of moderate-intensity exercise)	RMR × 1.55	2,277 kcal
Heavy training day (e.g., 2+ hr of high-intensity exercise)	RMR × 1.725	2,534 kcal
Intense training day (e.g., 2+ hr of nonstop high-intensity exercise)	RMR × 1.9	2,791 kcal

Energy Balance Versus Energy Availability

Energy balance is the difference between energy input and energy output. When body weight does not change over time, energy balance is 0 Calories per day because energy input minus energy output equals 0. If you consistently eat too much, energy balance becomes positive and you gain weight. If you consistently eat too little, energy balance becomes negative and you lose weight.

When energy input is restricted for prolonged periods (a few weeks or more of *energy deficiency*), RMR slows down as the body tries to compensate for reduced energy intake. When this happens, it becomes tougher to lose weight unless energy input continues to decrease. Athletes and fitness enthusiasts can experience energy deficiency as a result of *eating disorders* (e.g., anorexia nervosa), uninformed or misguided attempts to lose weight, unusual eating behaviors (often referred to as *disordered eating*, including fasting, laxatives, and induced vomiting), or an unintentional failure to eat enough.

Energy availability is a simple concept based on simple arithmetic: The difference between energy input and physical activity energy expenditure equals energy availability, the amount of energy that is available to meet the body's remaining

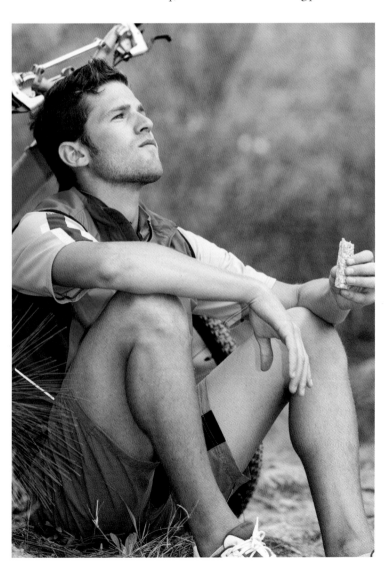

needs for energy. Here is one example using the hypothetical female volleyball player. If she consumes 2,356 Calories (kcal) on one day and expends 856 Calories during her training, her energy availability would be 2,356 − 856 = 1,500 Calories. For this particular day, the athlete would be in an energy deficit because her estimated energy needs in order to meet her RMR and basic daily activities (RMR × 1.2; see the calculations in table 7.3) is 1,856 Calories. If this pattern continued, the athlete would be in a state of energy deficiency and at possible risk for menstrual irregularities, loss of bone mineral content, and impaired performance in training and competition.

Calculating energy availability can be a useful tool in helping clients and athletes make informed decisions about strategies for weight loss and weight gain (see table 7.4). However, to have confidence in those calculations, you have to have an accurate idea of a person's typical daily energy input (in kcal/day), energy output (in kcal/day), body weight (in kg), and at least an approximation of fat-free mass (FFM, in kg). FFM is used in the calculations to represent the energy needs of the most metabolically active tissues of the body.

In working with athletes and fitness enthusiasts, it is important to be familiar with two additional terms: *relative energy deficit in sports* (RED-S) and the f*emale athlete triad*. RED-S refers to negative health and performance consequences of prolonged low energy availability in athletes and other physically active people. Those consequences include reproductive issues, poor bone health, reduced RMR, loss of muscle mass and strength, reduced training capacity, and poorer competitive performance. The female athlete triad is a term used to describe menstrual dysfunction, loss of bone mineral content, and disordered eating. Clients and athletes who have ongoing issues with maintaining a healthy body weight are best served by a specialist, such as a Registered Dietitian/Nutritionist (RDN), who can create individualized programs to address specific issues.

TABLE 7.4 **Calculating Energy Availability to Recommend Strategies for Weight Loss and Gain**

Goal	Evaluate risk of energy deficiency	Safely lose weight	Maintain or gain weight
Calorie intake	<30 kcal/kg FFM/day	30-45 kcal/kg FFM/day	>45 kcal/kg FFM/day
Example	122 lb female high school cross-country runner consumes 2,200 kcal/day and expends 950 kcal/day in training. She wants to maintain her current weight but struggles during some training sessions and races.	192 lb 46-year-old male recreational basketball player consumes 3,460 kcal/day and expends 625 kcal/day in fitness training and basketball games. He wants to lose weight to improve his long-term health and increase his quickness on the court.	212 lb 16-year-old high school male football player wants to gain weight but has been having a difficult time doing so. He typically consumes 4,300 kcal/day and expends 1,200 kcal/day during weightlifting and team practice sessions.
Energy availability	2,200 − 950 = 1,150 kcal/day. She has 16.5% body fat, so her FFM = 122 − (122 × .165) = 102 lb (46.4 kg).	3,460 − 625 = 2,835 kcal/day. He has 22.3% body fat, so his FFM = 192 − (192 × .223) = 149 lb (67.8 kg).	4,300 − 1,200 = 3,100 kcal/day. He has 14.4% body fat, so his FFM = 212 − (212 × .14) = 182 lb (82.9 kg).
Lowest estimated energy availability	30 × 46.4 = 1,390 kcal to meet daily nonexercise needs. This value > current energy availability of 1,150 kcal/day.	30 × 67.8 = 2,034 kcal to meet daily nonexercise needs. This value < current energy availability of 2,835 kcal/day.	45 × 82.9 = 3,729 kcal to meet daily nonexercise needs. This value > current energy availability of 3,100 kcal/day.
Recommendation	She is at risk of performance and health consequences of energy deficiency. She should increase energy input or reduce training load so that energy availability exceeds 1,400 kcal/day.	He could reduce energy intake by no more than 500 kcal/day and safely lose weight without being in danger of energy deficiency.	He should increase energy intake by at least 650 kcal/day to begin to gain weight.

Why Do Some People Have Difficulty Losing Weight?

In one sense, losing weight can be as easy as moving more and eating less. For some people it *is* that easy. After all, the laws of thermodynamics can't be broken: If you consistently ingest fewer calories than you expend, you will lose weight over time. Yet for some people, moving more and eating less do not have the same satisfying results. In fact, compared to people who are on an identical regimen of exercise and diet, they don't lose much weight at all. Why is that? Some of the factors that affect weight loss are summarized in figure 7.5, and the following sections discuss in more detail some of the variation that occurs among individuals. It is important to remember that losing weight and then maintaining that weight loss often require two different approaches. Losing weight is best accomplished by an emphasis on reducing caloric intake, while an emphasis on increased physical activity appears best for maintaining that weight loss.

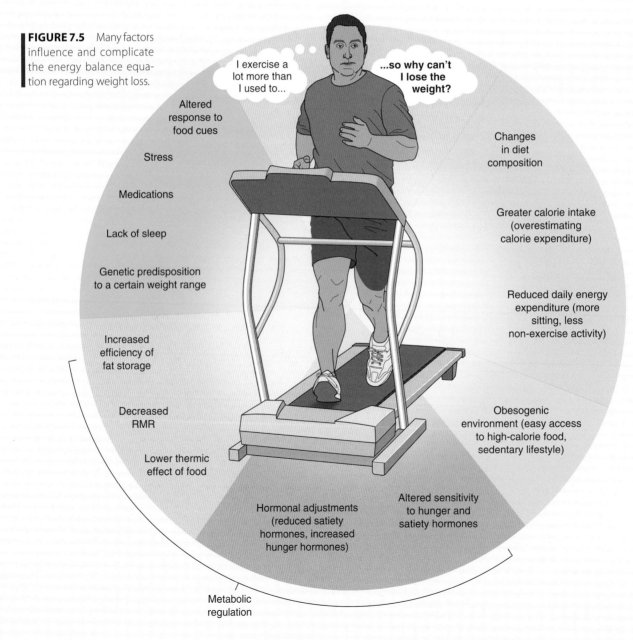

FIGURE 7.5 Many factors influence and complicate the energy balance equation regarding weight loss.

Genetics

Genes are pesky things. Some scientists think that genes determine body weight and make futile any attempt to establish a new body weight outside of a fairly narrow gene-determined range. Other scientists agree that genetics plays a role in body weight but not as the sole determining factor. Otherwise, how do you explain people who lose hundreds of pounds and maintain their new lower weight for decades? The current thinking is that genetics does play a role in predisposing some people to obesity, with physical activity and diet being the predominant factors in determining the rate and extent of weight gain. To be clear, once a person becomes obese, it is very difficult—but not impossible—to establish a healthier body weight.

Homeostatic Compensation

This sounds more complicated than it is. The thinking on homeostatic compensation is that your body establishes a set point for body weight, and that attempts to alter body weight provoke compensations to counter those attempts.

Here's a simple example: People who introduce exercise into their daily routine in an attempt to lose weight are often frustrated by the slow pace of weight loss. Research shows that when people begin to exercise regularly, they often increase their food intake and decrease their physical activity during the rest of the day. In addition, people on very-low-calorie diets often struggle to lose weight as the body tries to compensate for low energy intake by reducing RMR.

Consistently undereating decreases resting metabolic rate (RMR), the thermic effect of food (TEF), the energy cost of movement (due to weight loss), nonexercise activity thermogenesis (NEAT; posture, fidgeting), and satiety hormones (e.g., leptin, insulin, cholecystokinin), while hunger hormones (e.g., neuropeptide Y, ghrelin) are increased. In other words, undereating results in compensatory metabolic and behavioral responses that combine to work against weight loss. Those responses do not make it impossible to lose weight, but they can make it more challenging to do so.

Hormones

The neuroendocrine system (brain, central nervous system, hormones) plays an important role in the regulation of hunger and satiety. Eating provokes the release of dozens if not hundreds of hormones from the brain, gut, pancreas, liver, and other organs, creating a rich mix of signals that influence feelings of hunger and satiety. Some people may be more sensitive to those signals than others, and that higher sensitivity means that hunger is turned off sooner, so they eat less and don't gain weight.

Performance Nutrition Spotlight

Rapid weight loss can be achieved with low-calorie (800–1,200 kcal/day) and very-low-calorie (no more than 800 kcal/day) diets, but such severe energy restriction cannot be sustained for long and results in a decrease in resting metabolic rate, making weight loss more difficult. For effective long-term fat loss, a slower but steady rate of weight loss caused by modest calorie restriction (a reduction of between 250 and 500 kcal/day) and increased physical activity is the best way to go.

Undereating and overeating produce wide variations in weight loss and gain. For example, when a group of people overeat by 1,000 Calories (kcal) per day, the actual energy balance might vary from 100 to 700 Calories per day. Resistance to fat gain is explained by increases in NEAT, TEF, and energy expenditure.

What's the Best Way to Lose Fat but Protect Muscle Mass?

In chapter 6, you learned that muscle is very plastic; it quickly adapts to the stress placed on it and even more quickly loses those adaptations when the stress is removed. Adding muscle mass requires the right type of exercise and the right type of diet with an emphasis on consuming enough energy (calories) to increase or maintain muscle protein content. Along with adequate energy, muscles require carbohydrate, protein, and water for recovery, repair, and adaptation. Diets that restrict energy intake too severely run the risk of promoting muscle loss along with fat loss.

Clients and athletes who want to lose fat weight but maintain or increase muscle mass have to be careful about how much they restrict their energy intake. Large drops in energy intake (e.g., a reduction of 1,000 kcal/day) will definitely result in short-term weight loss, but some of that weight loss will be due to a loss in the size of muscle cells. When energy intake is restricted, muscle cells break down contractile proteins to produce energy (ATP) and are unable to repair or replace damaged proteins.

A very low caloric intake (e.g., 1,200 kcal/day or fewer) in adults provokes a compensatory decrease in RMR as the body tries to reduce its energy needs to cope with inadequate daily energy intake. Not surprisingly, a reduced RMR makes it tougher to lose weight, which is one of the reasons experts recommend a sustained weight loss of 1 to 2 pounds (0.5-1 kg) per week as a result of moderate energy intake restriction (a reduction of between 250 and 500 kcal/day) and an increase in daily energy expenditure.

Smaller drops in energy intake (e.g., eating 250-500 fewer kcal per day) result in slower rates of weight loss. Faster responses occur when exercise is used to increase energy expenditure with little or no decrease in energy intake. For example, if a person needs 2,500 Calories (kcal) per day to maintain current body weight, weight loss will occur if energy intake is reduced to 1,500 Calories per day. Weight loss will also occur and muscle mass will be better protected if the person increases energy output by 500 Calories per day along with establishing a modest decrease (about 250 fewer kcal per day) in energy input. When daily energy intake is restricted, increasing the protein content of the diet and continuing daily exercise is associated with greater weight loss, more fat loss, and less loss of lean tissue.

People who successfully lose large amounts of weight and keep it off have some things in common: Most eat breakfast every day. Most weigh themselves at least once each week. Most watch less than two hours of TV daily. And most exercise about an hour each day.

Performance Nutrition Spotlight

Research demonstrates that loss of muscle protein resulting from severe energy restriction can be reduced by increasing the amount of protein in the diet to 1.6 to 2.4 grams per kilogram per day (0.7-1.1 g/lb/day), more than twice the recommendation for protein intake in sedentary people.

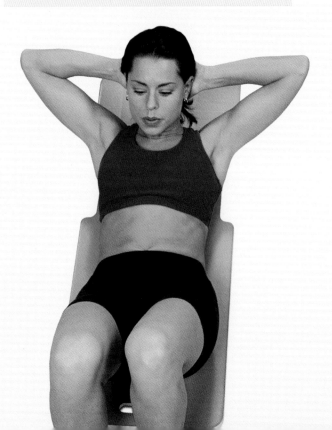

Aiming to lose fat weight at a gradual pace (i.e., 1 to 2 lb, or 0.5 to 1 kg, of body weight per week) reduces the chance of regaining the weight while also reducing the potentially negative impact on exercise and sport performance. Furthermore, a slow but steady pace of weight loss minimizes the loss of both muscle and water. Losing weight at a more rapid pace means losing muscle mass and becoming dehydrated, two negative consequences that impair both health and performance. Although it is possible to increase muscle mass during times of weight loss, muscle mass can only be maximized during times of energy balance. For athletes or people who are already active, maintaining or increasing physical activity energy expenditure while modestly reducing energy intake by 250 to 500 Calories (kcal) per day is usually enough to promote a loss of 1 to 2 pounds (0.5-1 kg) of fat each week. Some people scoff at the idea of losing only 1 pound (0.5 kg) of fat per week, but they fail to recognize that at that rate, weight loss would add up to 52 pounds (23 kg) in a year!

Compared to males at any relative body mass index (BMI) value, twice as many females perceive themselves as overweight. For example, a woman at the 50th percentile for BMI (i.e., 50% of women have a higher BMI and 50% have a lower BMI) is twice as likely as a man at the 50th percentile for BMI to feel overweight and to be engaged in trying to lose weight.

What's the Best Way to Lose Abdominal Fat?

This is one question that will always be asked, in large part because many people don't understand the basics of fat loss. The way in which fat is stored varies between sexes and among people. Many females deposit fat on their hips, leading to pear-shaped *gynoid obesity*. Many males tend to deposit fat in the abdominal region, leading to apple-shaped *android obesity*. Obviously not all overweight women are shaped like pears, nor are all overweight men shaped like apples. There is a wide range within the sexes in how fat is deposited throughout the body. That wide range also determines how fat is lost from the body. For example, a person who is genetically predisposed to accumulating fat in the abdominal area will first notice fat loss in that area, even though fat is being lost from fat cells throughout the person's entire body.

Loss of excess abdominal fat is the result of the loss of fatty acids from fat cells throughout the body, including the abdomen. Doing endless crunches and planks will strengthen the abdominal muscles and improve the chances that a six-pack will eventually emerge, but those exercises will not spot-reduce abdominal fat. Fat loss is enhanced by increasing energy output and reducing energy input. It's just impossible to stray far from the energy balance equation!

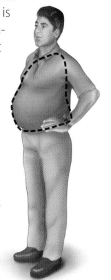 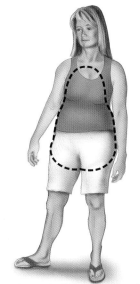

Upper body (android) obesity   Lower body (gynoid) obesity

Adapted by permission from W.L. Kenney, J.H. Wilmore, and D.L. Costill, *Physiology of Sport and Exercise*, 7th ed. (Champaign, IL: Human Kinetics, 2020), 561.

What Is the Fat-Burning Zone?

From a scientific standpoint, there is no single fat-burning zone. Your body is constantly burning fat; the amount of fat being burned (oxidized to produce ATP) rises and falls depending mostly on your physical activity. The popular notion of the fat-burning zone is that there is a range of exercise intensity (often linked to exercise heart rate) that maximizes the amount of fat being burned during exercise. But as shown in figure 7.6, the total energy expended during exercise, not the source of that energy, is most important for weight loss. Also note that the amount of fat oxidized *during* exercise is often very small; the total number of calories expended during the day (total energy expenditure) determines how much fat is lost over time.

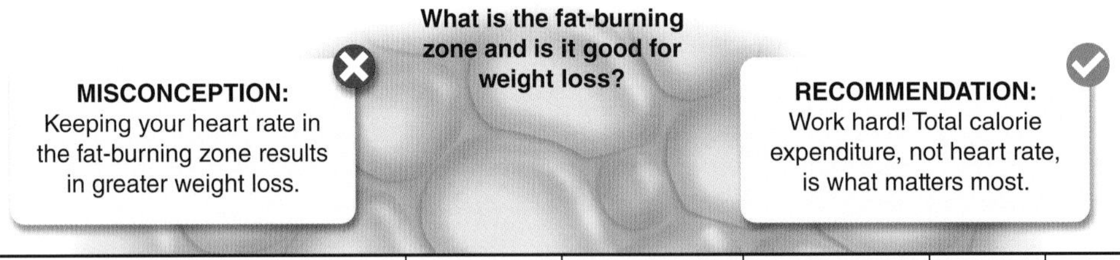

What is the fat-burning zone and is it good for weight loss?

MISCONCEPTION: Keeping your heart rate in the fat-burning zone results in greater weight loss.

RECOMMENDATION: Work hard! Total calorie expenditure, not heart rate, is what matters most.

		Intensity	$\dot{V}O_2$ (L/min)	% kcal from carbohydrate	% kcal from fat	kcal/hour
If you exercise at 50% of your maximal heart rate about 50% of ATP production will come from fat oxidation and 50% from glucose oxidation. 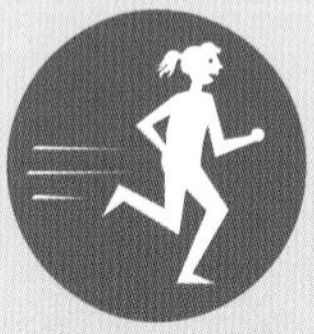		50% HR$_{max}$	1.50	50%	50%	440
Increase your intensity to 75% HR$_{max}$, and your fat oxidation will drop to 33% of ATP production. That drop might seem counterproductive to fat loss, but it isn't. Energy expenditure is greater at higher exercise intensities and that number is what counts in overall energy balance (or energy availability). 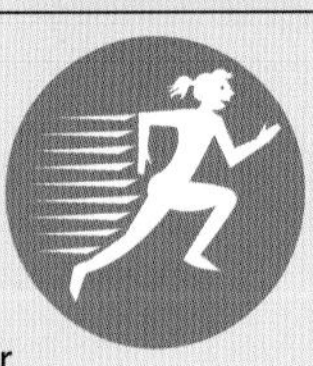		75% HR$_{max}$	2.25	67%	33%	664

In most cases, oxidation from fat stores during exercise = 1 oz/hour

FIGURE 7.6   The fat-burning zone is meaningless for weight loss because overall energy expenditure and energy intake are what determine fat loss over time.

Adapted by permission from W.L. Kenney, J.H. Wilmore, and D.L. Costill, *Physiology of Sport and Exercise,* 7th ed. (Champaign, IL: Human Kinetics, 2020), 567.

Does Consuming Calories During Exercise Defeat the Weight-Loss Purpose of Exercise?

Short answer: No. Look at figure 7.7 for an extreme example. It's easy to understand why people believe that if their goal is to lose weight, they shouldn't consume calories during exercise—a time when they are working hard to expend calories. Yet, research shows very clearly that ingesting carbohydrate calories (energy) during a workout is often associated with an increase in energy expenditure (more calories burned) because the exercising muscles have an additional fuel source and can work harder. Keep in mind that overall energy expenditure during the day—the total of physical activity energy expenditure and nonexercise activity thermogenesis, or NEAT—determines total energy output.

Performance Nutrition Spotlight

Walking is a great way to expend energy and can help you lose weight. Some research shows that chewing gum during walks actually increases the calories burned, perhaps because walking cadence increases to keep pace with chewing. The increase in calories burned is small, but could be meaningful over many months of daily walking.

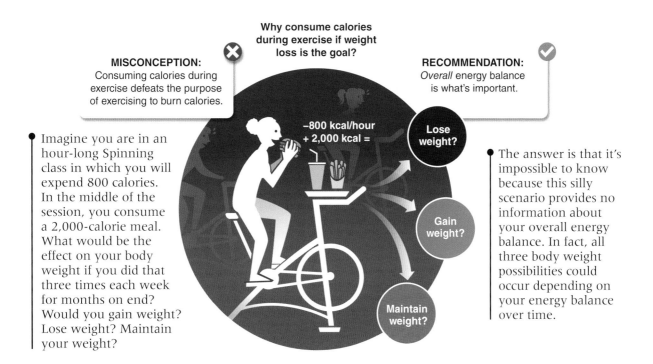

Why consume calories during exercise if weight loss is the goal?

MISCONCEPTION: Consuming calories during exercise defeats the purpose of exercising to burn calories.

RECOMMENDATION: *Overall* energy balance is what's important.

−800 kcal/hour + 2,000 kcal =

Lose weight?

Gain weight?

Maintain weight?

Imagine you are in an hour-long Spinning class in which you will expend 800 calories. In the middle of the session, you consume a 2,000-calorie meal. What would be the effect on your body weight if you did that three times each week for months on end? Would you gain weight? Lose weight? Maintain your weight?

The answer is that it's impossible to know because this silly scenario provides no information about your overall energy balance. In fact, all three body weight possibilities could occur depending on your energy balance over time.

FIGURE 7.7 Ingesting calories during exercise in the form of sports drinks, carbohydrate gels, energy bars, or any other food source will not make it more difficult to lose fat. Weight loss depends on overall energy balance, not just the energy (calories) consumed on a specific occasion.

Will Exercising While Fasting Increase Fat Oxidation and Weight Loss?

There is no doubt that fasting causes the body to limit its use of carbohydrate and rely more on the oxidation of fatty acids to produce ATP. So fasting does cause an increase in fat oxidation (fat burning). Similar increases in fat oxidation occur when consuming a high-fat, low-carbohydrate diet. But as shown in figure 7.8, fasting reduces the body's use of carbohydrate during exercise and consequently its ability to maintain power output. That's not a good thing because reduced power also means reduced energy expenditure—fewer calories are burned.

Although some people believe that high-fat diets are good for appetite control, fat is actually the weakest macronutrient at producing satiety and at increasing its own oxidation. True high-fat diets deplete muscle and liver glycogen, leading to the loss of water molecules that are normally stored with glycogen. Water loss, not fat loss, explains most of the rapid weight loss that occurs in the early stages of such dieting.

Will training in a fasted state or when avoiding carbohydrates enhance muscles' ability to burn fat?

MISCONCEPTION:
Training fasted ramps up fat burning.

RECOMMENDATION:
It does, but performance suffers. You are likely to work out harder and burn more calories when carbohydrate stores are normal.

Fasting or low-carbohydrate, high-fat diets lead to

• Enhanced fat oxidation
• Impaired carbohydrate oxidation
• Lower training workloads
• Altered immune response
• Poorer performance

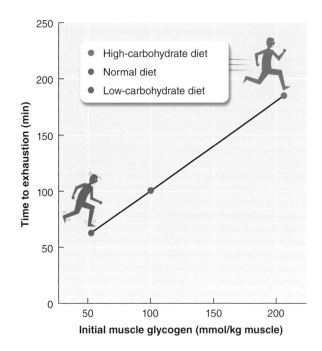

FIGURE 7.8 Fasting and low-carbohydrate diets do increase the amount of fat the body oxidizes (burns), but these practices also reduce the carbohydrate available to muscle, which shortens the time to exhaustion and limits the ability to train at high levels.

Adapted by permission from W.L. Kenney, J.H. Wilmore, and D.L. Costill, *Physiology of Sport and Exercise*, 7th ed. (Champaign, IL: Human Kinetics, 2020), 389.

Chapter Summary

- Weight loss occurs whenever energy expenditure regularly exceeds energy intake for more than a few days.
- For most people, restricting energy intake is the most effective way to initiate weight loss and increased physical activity is the best way to maintain weight loss.
- Regular physical activity increases daily energy expenditure and is the major contributor to the energy deficit required for weight loss.
- Many athletes expend more than 1,000 kcal per day in training, so some fat loss is an almost inevitable outcome.
- The energy balance equation illustrates that weight loss will occur whenever there is an energy deficit sufficient to result in substantial oxidation of stored fat. There are many factors that complicate that simple picture and a reduced RMR is one of them.
- No one weight-loss diet is better than another. The most effective approach to weight loss is the one that can be maintained long-term with no ill effects on health or performance.

Review Questions

1. Explain the concept of energy balance.
2. Describe two reasons why some people have a difficult time losing fat weight even though they increase their physical activity.
3. Briefly detail the components of daily energy expenditure.
4. Explain how energy availability is important in determining the daily energy needs of athletes.
5. Discuss the fallacy of the fat-burning zone.

CHAPTER EIGHT

Training for Speed and Power

Objectives

- Understand the adaptations in muscles, connective tissues, and the nervous system related to improved speed and power.
- Appreciate how enhanced speed and power contribute to improved performance in all physical activities.
- Recognize the importance of metabolic flexibility as one benefit of speed and power training.

Speed and power are critical elements in all athletic events. Even for those uninterested in competition but desiring improved fitness, enhanced speed and power are unavoidable by-products of training. A football player tackling a ball-carrier, a wrestler shooting for a single-leg takedown, a volleyball player leaping for a spike, a gymnast executing a dismount, a swimmer exploding from the starting block, a basketball player sprinting down the court to get back on defense, and a javelin athlete on the final step before a throw all exhibit important combinations of speed and power. In those examples, it's easy to understand how improved speed and power are related to improved performance. But the same is true for a middle-aged woman newly enrolled in a fitness class, a recreational runner trying for a personal record in a 5K race, and a 74-year-old man working to regain leg strength after a hip replacement.

It's easy to understand why speed and power are important to athletes, and it's equally easy to understand why people interested in losing weight, improving muscle tone, or enhancing overall fitness would not think in terms of improving their speed and power as personal goals. Yet, all training programs influence speed and power, even when speed, power, and sport performance are of no interest to an individual.

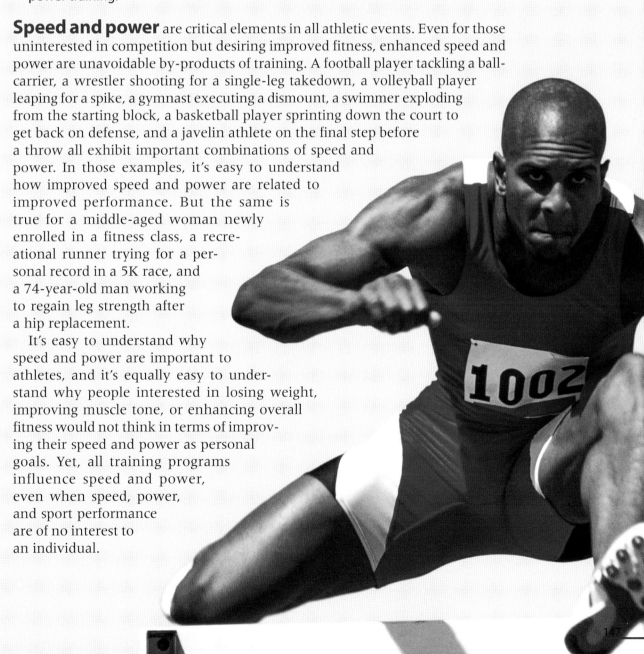

What Are Speed and Power?

Speed and power are inextricably linked because power is influenced by speed. You intuitively know what speed and power mean in the exercise and sport settings, but in a book like this one, it's good to begin with clear definitions of those terms (also see figure 8.1).

Speed is a measure of the rate of motion; in math terms, speed (S) is the distance (D) traveled divided by the time (T) it takes to travel that distance:

$$S = D / T$$

When you can cover the same or more distance in less time, you've become faster. Your speed has increased.

Power is a measure of the rate at which energy is transferred; mathematically, power (P) is force (F) multiplied by distance (D) and divided by time (T). In other words, power is a measure of how quickly a force can be moved:

$$P = (F \times D) / T$$

In this simple equation, force (F) can refer to body weight or to the weight of a barbell or the resistance setting on a piece of exercise equipment. Power is determined by the amount of force and the speed at which that force is applied or resisted. For example, a football player becomes more powerful as he becomes faster, provided his body weight has not decreased. Increased power is particularly important in football, weightlifting, throwing sports, and sprint events of any kind. Speed and power usually improve together with training, but there are times when it makes sense to be more concerned with improving speed even if power decreases. That's certainly the case in all timed events in running, swimming, and cycling when finishing first is the goal. Generally speaking, power increases as a person becomes faster, but there are occasions when an athlete needs to lose fat weight to increase speed. If the decrease in body weight (F in the power equation) falls more than the increase in speed (D / T), then power will drop slightly, but that's of little consequence if the goal of increasing speed has been achieved.

Power is not often considered important for marathon runners and other endurance athletes, but both speed and power are critical for all sports. Speed in large part determines power, and the ability to generate greater amounts of power is just as important for endurance athletes as it is for football players and athletes in other explosive sports. Although endurance athletes generate far less maximal power than sprint athletes, endurance athletes are able to maintain power output for long periods. Sprinters and endurance athletes all must improve speed and power in order to improve their performance. Well-designed training programs improve speed, power, and endurance capacity.

Even with interval training and fitness classes of any sort, as people become more fit, lose weight, and improve their skills, their speed and power will be positively affected. While that improvement should not be the only goal for recreational exercisers, it's important to keep in mind that all types of training influence speed and power.

Performance Nutrition Spotlight

Rinsing the mouth with a sugar solution can improve performance in events lasting less than 45 minutes, when there is not enough time for ingested carbohydrate to be absorbed and metabolized. Mouth rinsing during HIIT sessions is a good example of this practice.

Speed is a measure of the rate of motion.

Power is a measure of the rate at which energy is transferred.

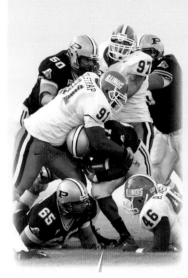
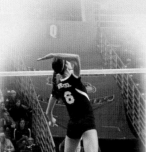
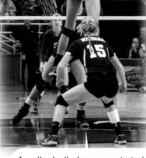
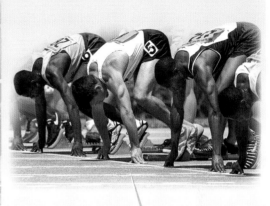

A 150-pound speedy halfback will not generate as much power when he hits the defensive line as will a slower 225-pound halfback. The heavier player has a slower rate of motion (speed) but a greater rate of energy transfer (power). If either athlete became faster, his power would increase. The same is true if either athlete gained muscle mass and maintained the same speed.

A volleyball player wants to be able to spike the ball more forcefully. Strength and skill training increase the muscle mass and strength in her shoulder and arm as well as the speed at which she hits the ball. Now the rate of her arm motion (speed) and the mass of her shoulder and arm have increased, resulting in a more powerful spike (increased rate of energy transfer).

A 100-meter sprinter dedicates himself to off-season strength training in an attempt to become faster. His training is successful as he adds 12 pounds of muscle and gains strength in all his lifts, especially in his upper body. But his initial times are disappointing, significantly slower than at the start of the previous season. In this case, the increase in body mass slowed his rate of motion (speed), even though his rate of energy transfer (power) may have remained the same.

FIGURE 8.1 Speed and power are important factors in all athletic pursuits, from short sprints to ultramarathons. The amount of power that the body generates during activity is related to speed of movement and the force (weight, also known as mass) being moved.

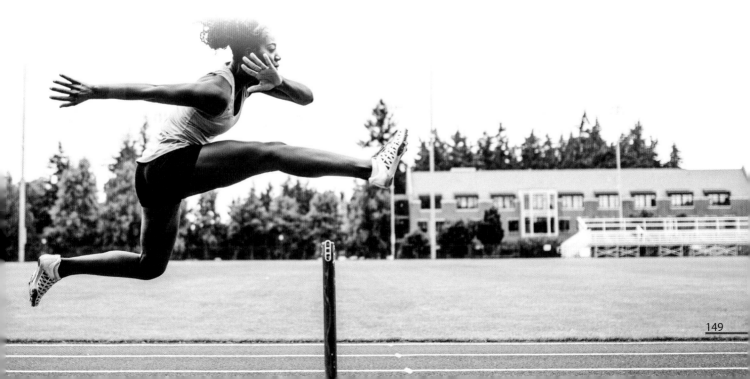

What Adaptations Are Needed to Improve Speed and Power?

Increasing speed and power requires that active muscle cells be able to produce ATP at a higher rate, sustain that production rate for a longer time, and generate more force in the process. In this case, *force* refers to the strength of each contraction. Recruiting more motor units helps in achieving those goals, as does increasing the myofibril content of muscle cells. All those adaptations are made possible by proper training.

Improving the capacity for exercise—any sort of exercise—requires the right stimulus (training) to provoke an optimal response (adaptation). Improvements in speed and power are no exception. Common sense combined with a little knowledge about training adaptations indicates that speed and power training should result in improvements in anaerobic ATP production along with increases in muscle strength and other changes needed to support a faster, more powerful athlete. Speed and power training results in a variety of adaptations that improve the capacity for high-intensity exercise.

Speed and power training is of obvious importance for athletes in sports that require brief, explosive movements; however, because of the interconnectedness of the energy systems, aerobic training is also relevant for all athletes. You learned that ATP is constantly being produced from anaerobic (PCr and glycolysis) and from aerobic (Krebs cycle, electron transport chain) processes. This is true at rest and during all types of physical activity; muscle cells simply adjust their reliance on the energy pathways based on how rapidly ATP must be produced. The ability of muscle cells to transition among the energy pathways is referred to as *metabolic flexibility*. For example, even though the average American football play lasts only about 6 seconds, there is an endurance (aerobic) component to those brief, explosive activities, as well as the recovery periods that follow, especially when the players are on the field for extended periods.

Sport training always involves a combination of aerobic and anaerobic ATP production. For example, shot putters require improved aerobic capacity to support their intense training sessions, even though during competition each effort lasts only a few seconds.

> An individual's genetics determines the upper limit of what training can accomplish, but no genes are linked strongly enough with performance to justify using genetics to predict athletic success.

Benefits of Speed and Power Training

- Stronger muscles
- Bigger muscles
- Greater ATP production
- Faster ATP production
- Greater and more synchronous motor unit recruitment
- Increased power
- Increased muscle fiber cross-sectional area
- Increased percentage of type II fibers
- Stronger connections between tendons and bones
- Stronger bones
- Faster reaction times
- Increased agility
- Improved skills at speed
- Greater ground reaction forces

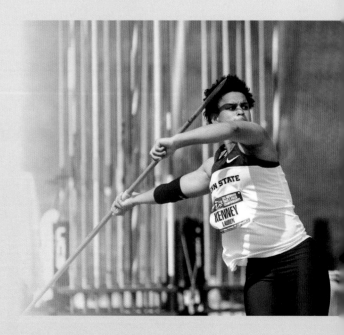

What Kinds of Training Improve Speed and Power?

The *principle of specificity* (see chapter 5 for a refresher) indicates that adaptations to training are specific to the mode and intensity of the training. Common sense dictates that if you want to improve speed in the 100-meter sprint, it would be silly to train like an endurance athlete. Fortunately, a variety of approaches that can be integrated into any training program can enhance speed and power.

Interval Training

Interval training has been a staple of elite athletes since at least the 1930s. Interval training intersperses exercise and rest in an endless variety of ways and can be used with any sport or physical pursuit; interval programs can be designed for everyone, from sprinters to ultraendurance athletes. One advantage of interval training is that it allows for repeated high-intensity efforts that help maximize the exercise stimulus and optimize training adaptations. Interspersing bouts of exercise with rest periods allows for higher exercise intensities than what can be sustained during continuous exercise. High exercise intensity is a greater stimulus to provoke training adaptations because of the increased demands on the cardiorespiratory system, the metabolic pathways required to produce ATP, the buffering systems needed to control metabolic acid buildup, the ability of the nervous system to recruit motor units, and the capacity to store and use carbohydrate and fat.

Performance Nutrition Spotlight

Consuming 20 to 40 grams of protein before bedtime will increase muscle protein synthesis during sleep, helping to increase muscle mass and strength over time. That protein can be from meat (beef, chicken, pork, poultry, etc.), fish, dairy, grains, nuts, beans, and seeds.

As you can see in the examples in the sidebars, the right combination of exercise intensity and rest (the work-to-rest ratio) depends on the athlete's fitness and training goals. There is no single work-to-rest ratio that is optimal; the design of interval training workouts should reflect the objective of the training session and the overall goal of the training program. Here are some examples of interval training:

- Jump rope 30 seconds on and 30 seconds off for 12 minutes
- Run 4 reps of 3 minutes on and 3 minutes off
- Cycle 20 seconds all-out and 2 minutes off; repeat 6 times
- Swim 12 × 100 yards every 90 seconds
- Run 6 stair sprints, 1 every 3 minutes

Circuit training is a form of interval training that usually involves a series of resistance and body-weight exercises (e.g., bench press, pull-up, biceps curl, leg extension, push-ups) with short rest intervals between each. Completion of all the exercises represents a circuit.

Fartlek training—also called speed-play training—was developed in Sweden in the late 1930s and is a hybrid of continuous training and interval training. In Fartlek training, continuous exercise at a sustainable intensity is periodically interrupted by bouts of high-intensity efforts typically lasting 30 seconds to 3 minutes.

Out-of-Shape Softball Player: Work-to-Rest Ratio

Goal: Improve speed and agility. Reduce risk of knee injury.

The objective of this sample 45-minute interval training session is to practice proper running and jumping mechanics while completing exercises designed to improve quadriceps, hamstring, and core strength and stamina. As fitness and movement skills improve, the number of reps and sets can gradually increase and the rest intervals can decrease.

- Warm-up: 15-minute combination of walking, jogging, running, stretching.
- 3 sets of 30-yard jog, run, sprint, 1 every 30 seconds. Rest as needed.
- 4 reps of 30-second body planks: front, right, front, left, with 30-second rest between each.
- 4 reps of 10-yard agility squares: side shuffle right, backpedal, side shuffle left, sprint forward. One square every 30 seconds or rest as needed.
- 8 depth jumps, each from 1-foot height with soft, stable landing.
- 10 reps of stability-ball leg curls.
- Repeat 4 reps of 10-yard agility squares: side shuffle right, backpedal, side shuffle left, sprint forward. Rest as needed.
- Cool-down.

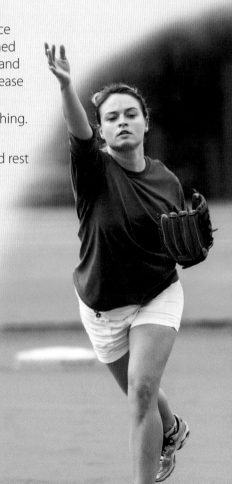

In recent years, research has shown that comparatively brief sessions of *high-intensity interval training* (HIIT) is effective in improving aerobic and anaerobic fitness with minimal time commitment. HIIT sessions are designed to provoke maximal intracellular signaling through brief (e.g., 10-30 sec), repeated bouts of all-out efforts. For athletes interested in improving speed and power, periodic HIIT workouts make great sense. For anyone desiring to improve their overall fitness, HIIT sessions produce significant fitness benefits for a minimal investment of time (but maximal investment of effort).

The principle of specificity is still a valid concept for sport training in that the bulk of training time should be devoted to sport-specific skill and fitness development. Until recently, the prevailing thinking was that endurance athletes should train primarily with long-duration bouts of exercise to mimic the demands of their endurance sport. Although interval training has always been a staple of endurance training, very short-duration, high-intensity interval training was not often used as a way to build endurance capacity. However, research has shown that HIIT can benefit endurance performance. Research conducted on trained and untrained individuals shows that HIIT produces adaptations commonly linked with endurance training, such as increased concentrations of oxidative (aerobic) enzymes in muscle cells.[*]

[*]Reference: Gibala, M.J., McGee, S.L. 2018. Metabolic adaptations to short-term high-intensity interval training: a little pain for a lot of gain? *Exercise and Sport Sciences Reviews.* 36(2):58-63.

Collegiate Soccer Player: Work-to-Rest Ratio

Goal: Improve end-of-game stamina and agility.

The objective of this sample 60-minute interval training session conducted in a fitness facility is to challenge the core and leg muscles before completing an agility drill and high-intensity sprints. Improved performances on the agility drill and high-intensity sprints at the end of the workout signal when to increase the reps and sets for the preceding exercises.

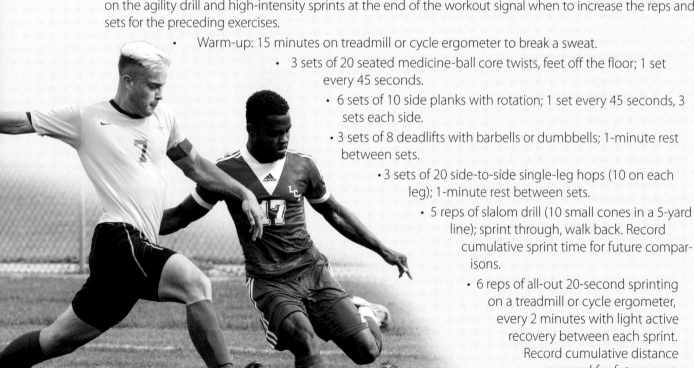

- Warm-up: 15 minutes on treadmill or cycle ergometer to break a sweat.
- 3 sets of 20 seated medicine-ball core twists, feet off the floor; 1 set every 45 seconds.
- 6 sets of 10 side planks with rotation; 1 set every 45 seconds, 3 sets each side.
- 3 sets of 8 deadlifts with barbells or dumbbells; 1-minute rest between sets.
- 3 sets of 20 side-to-side single-leg hops (10 on each leg); 1-minute rest between sets.
- 5 reps of slalom drill (10 small cones in a 5-yard line); sprint through, walk back. Record cumulative sprint time for future comparisons.
- 6 reps of all-out 20-second sprinting on a treadmill or cycle ergometer, every 2 minutes with light active recovery between each sprint. Record cumulative distance covered for future comparisons.

HIIT Examples

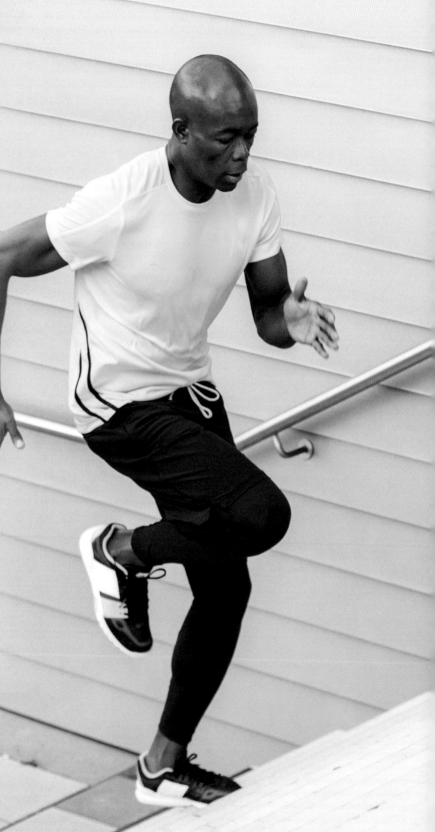

Example 1
- 5-minute warm-up
- 30-second all-out cycling
- 3.5-minute rest
- Repeat 5 times

Example 2
- 3-minute treadmill warm-up walk
- 3-minute fast walk
- 3-minute recovery walk
- Repeat 4 times

Example 3
- 3-minute warm-up jog
- 30-second run
- 20-second faster run
- 10-second sprint
- 3-minute walk/jog
- Repeat 3 times

Benefits
- Increased endurance capacity
- Increased maximal power
- Increased strength
- Increased muscle oxidative capacity
- Increased muscle glycogen
- Reduced lactate production
- Increased muscle mitochondrial biogenesis
- Increased intracellular signaling
- Increased carbohydrate and fat oxidation
- Increased $\dot{V}O_{2max}$
- Improved blood vessel membrane function
- Improved blood glucose control
- Increased size of type II muscle cells
- Increased glycolytic enzymes
- Increased ATP/PCr enzymes

Determining Intensity for Anaerobic Training

Training intensity during workouts is typically monitored using heart rate, metabolic equivalents (METs), or rating of perceived exertion (RPE; see table 8.1). A well-designed training program includes activities conducted at varying intensities, and usually only a small portion (e.g., 10-20%) of the weekly training load is conducted at very high intensity. As an athlete's or client's fitness improves, training intensity will naturally increase. Outside of a laboratory setting, monitoring training intensity is an imprecise science. Unlike endurance training where a $\dot{V}O_{2max}$ test in a laboratory setting is a universally accepted method for assessing aerobic capacity, there is less agreement on testing for anaerobic power. The Wingate test (30-second all-out cycling), oxygen-deficit testing, and critical-power testing can be used to measure and assess changes in anaerobic power, although each of those tests is best accomplished in an exercise science laboratory.

Heart rate can be tracked during a standard bout of exercise to assess changes in aerobic fitness. Changes in heart rate are related to changes in oxygen consumption, the gold-standard measure of exercise intensity. Monitoring just heart rate is not very valuable unless you know the individual's maximum heart rate. Maximum heart rate can be measured during a progressive exercise test to exhaustion, or it can be estimated from equations developed in laboratory experiments. There are numerous formulas for estimating maximal heart rate (HR_{max}), the basis for establishing heart rate ranges (zones) that correspond to various exercise intensities.

Monitoring heart rate can be a gauge of exercise intensity, but it is important to keep in mind that heart rate is affected by dehydration, heat, illness, and other stresses that can cause misleading heart rate responses. For example, if an athlete is accustomed to training in a heart rate zone of 135 to 145 beats per minute (bpm) during endurance training, simply being dehydrated can increase heart rate by 10 beats per minute or more, making it appear as though the athlete is working harder than she actually is.

Metabolic equivalents (METs) are often used in clinical settings such as cardiac rehabilitation and occupational therapy facilities to help monitor and control exercise intensity after heart surgery or injury. Exercise programs for older adults can incorporate the use of METs as a way to gauge progress in restoring or improving the physical capacity required for the tasks of everyday living.

Most people intuitively rely on some variation of the rating of perceived exertion (RPE) scale to align their exercise intensity with how they feel during a workout or competition. Educating athletes and clients about the proper use of a simple RPE scale (see table 8.1) can be useful in establishing the intensity of effort suited to various tasks. Of course, RPE scales rely on the individual's assessment of and comfort with physical effort, so differences among people introduce variability in their responses. As an example, if an instructor of a Spinning class asks the class to adjust the resistance on the bike to a "moderately heavy exertion" level (e.g., RPE of 5 on a scale of 1 to 10), there will be a large variability among class members in the actual resistance settings on their bikes. Those who are diligent about their training will follow the instructions, while those who decide not to work as hard have that option. Motivated and experienced athletes and clients are accustomed to pushing themselves and adjusting their efforts to fit the demands of training and competition.

Research indicates that improving core stability and core strength does not appear to be linked to improved sport performance.

TABLE 8.1 Rating of Perceived Exertion (RPE) Is an Easy Way for Athletes to Gauge Exercise Intensity

1	No exertion	Resting
2	Very light exertion	Easy to maintain without much effort
3	Light exertion	Takes a little effort, but could continue for an hour or more
4		
5	Moderately heavy exertion	Faster breathing and heart rate, but can talk
6	Heavy exertion	Can talk in short sentences but can't maintain this effort for long
7		
8	Extremely heavy exertion	Breathing too hard to speak
9	Almost maximal exertion	Gasping for breath
10	Maximal exertion	Can't work any harder or go more than 30 seconds

Largely adapted from the general principles of the OMNI scale found in A.C. Utter et al., "Validation of the Adult OMNI Scale of Perceived Exertion for Walking/Running Exercise," *Medicine Science and Sports Exercise* 36, no. 10 (2004): 1776-1780.

Plyometric Training

Plyometric training is often a focus for athletes who want to increase power and speed. Stretching a muscle before it contracts adds to the force and power of the contraction. Virtually all human movements—especially sport movements—involve a combination of eccentric (lengthening) and concentric (shortening) contractions. Plyometric exercises such as box jumping and bounding help athletes take better advantage of stretch–shortening movements. The likely effects of plyometric training are described in figure 8.2.

Eccentric training can enhance muscular strength and power by increasing muscle mass and the rate at which muscles develop force as well as increasing the length of muscle fasciculi and the number of sarcomeres in type II (fast-twitch) muscle fibers.

Keep in mind that the eccentric contractions that are part of plyometric training increase the risk of muscle damage, soreness, and injury to other tissues, so athletes and clients should do such exercise sparingly and at low intensity until they become accustomed to the movements.

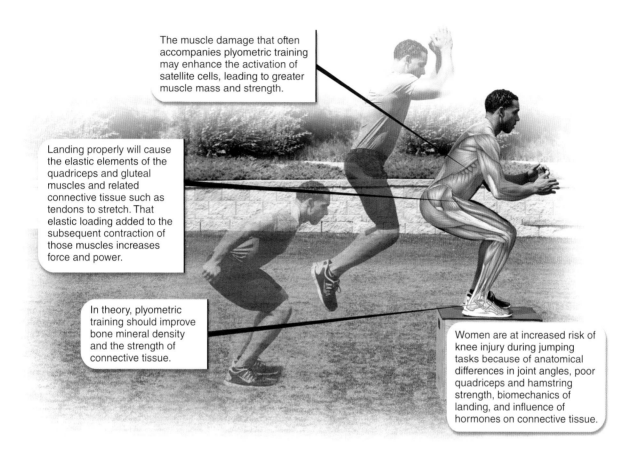

The muscle damage that often accompanies plyometric training may enhance the activation of satellite cells, leading to greater muscle mass and strength.

Landing properly will cause the elastic elements of the quadriceps and gluteal muscles and related connective tissue such as tendons to stretch. That elastic loading added to the subsequent contraction of those muscles increases force and power.

In theory, plyometric training should improve bone mineral density and the strength of connective tissue.

Women are at increased risk of knee injury during jumping tasks because of anatomical differences in joint angles, poor quadriceps and hamstring strength, biomechanics of landing, and influence of hormones on connective tissue.

FIGURE 8.2 Plyometric training triggers several adaptations, including increased ability to generate power.

Ballistic Training

Traditional strength training movement is done at slow speeds compared to movement speeds in many sports. In addition, considerable time in weightlifting movement is devoted to decelerating the weight toward the end of the range of motion. *Ballistic training* uses throwing, jumping, and striking movements to avoid that deceleration and thereby augment neuromuscular power. The intent of ballistic training is to increase motor unit recruitment with the goal of producing higher rates of force development. Ballistic training can be done with various loads and is perhaps best introduced after athletes or clients have established sound strength training skills. Examples of ballistic movements include medicine ball throws, jump squats (with or without added weight), and explosive push-ups.

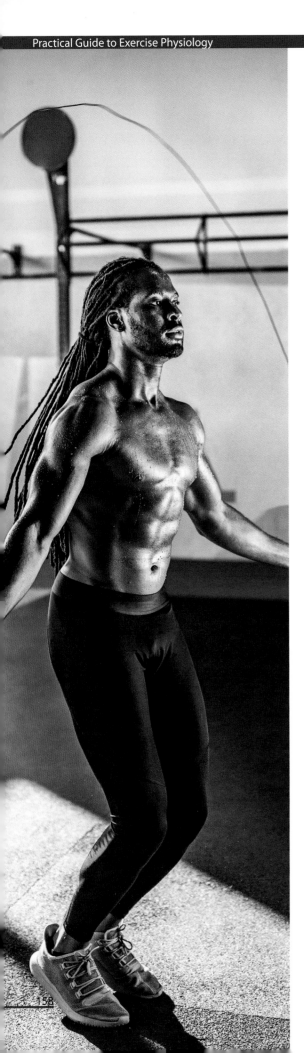

Cross-Training

Cross-training—training for more than one sport or activity at a time—provides variety to workouts. It also develops complementary new skills and promotes training adaptations that might otherwise be missed in sport-specific training. There appears to be little risk in cross-training provided it does not detract from time spent developing sport-specific skills and fitness. An example of an athlete using cross-training is a triathlete who has to train in swimming, cycling, and running, often combined with strength training and flexibility exercises. Other examples include wrestlers and swimmers who run and cycle, football and basketball players who participate in aerobic dance classes, and ice hockey players who circuit train.

Proper cross-training should introduce mental and physical variety and complement the overall intent of the training program. Also, effective cross-training should have a well-defined purpose. It makes no sense for basketball players to participate in aerobic dance unless the anticipated outcomes are clearly defined ahead of time and match the training needs of the athletes. Here are a few things to keep in mind when planning how to integrate cross-training into an athlete's training schedule:

- Adaptations to HIIT most resemble the changes in muscle and the cardiovascular system seen with endurance training. An advantage of HIIT is that muscle strength and power, along with improvements in anaerobic capacity, also occur.

- Strength benefits can be blunted by too much endurance training. Research indicates that strength development can be blunted somewhat by concurrent endurance training, something to keep in mind when designing training programs for individuals for whom strength development is the primary training objective. As an example, an athlete who has had a leg immobilized for weeks because of injury will have lost muscle mass and strength. Introducing endurance training too soon in the return-to-play training program will risk blunting strength development.

- Cross-training can result in improvements in endurance, strength, and power that are complementary to sport performance.

- Cross-training can also help reduce the risk of overtraining and overuse injuries in susceptible athletes and can be part of a return-to-play training plan after injury.

Adaptations to HIIT most resemble the changes in muscle and the cardiovascular system seen with endurance training. An advantage of HIIT is that improvements in muscle strength, power, and glycolytic capacity also occur.

What Does a Speed and Power Training Session Look Like?

Table 8.2 provides an example of a short speed and power training session. As with all types of training sessions, there are endless ways to mix the elements of speed and power training to create variety and maximize the training stimulus.

Improvements in performance of vertical jump occur with a combination of plyometric and resistance training to improve strength, power, coordination, and the elastic elements associated with jumping.

TABLE 8.2 **Sample 35-Minute Speed and Power Training Session**

Phase	Goals	Exercise	Time or reps
Warm-up	Increase heart rate, breathing, muscle temperature in preparation for harder efforts	Jump rope	2 min
Plyo box • Circuit format × 2; 30 sec recovery between sets • From a plyo box or stand; explosive but controlled movements	Begin w/ plyo box movements to continue to warm the body and prepare for maximal speed efforts	Step up to reverse lunge	6 reps each
		Depth jump to vertical jump	6 reps
Sprint efforts	Post sprint, keep recovery ratio at least 2:1 (of sprint effort)	Sprint repeats × 4	Turf 40-60 yd or Treadmill 20-30 sec (time accounts for belt to speed up on treadmill)
Med ball • Circuit format × 2; 30 sec recovery between sets • Explosive & lengthen through movements	Intersperse core, throwing, and eccentric movements with sprinting to improve speed and power	Sit-up to toss	12 reps each
		Power slams (to floor)	12 reps
Sprint efforts • Use round 1 as your benchmark to push yourself	Post sprint, keep recovery ratio at least 2:1 (of sprint effort)	Sprint repeats × 4	Turf 40-60 yd or Treadmill 20-30 sec (time accounts for belt to speed up on treadmill)
Strength & conditioning Dumbbell or barbell	Improve upper- and lower-body strength, explosiveness, and stamina	Front squat	6 reps
		Reverse lunge w/ overhead press	6 reps each
		Calf raise	12 reps

Sample workout by Kelly Schnell, BS, CSCS, ACSM-CPT, Inspyr Studios, Arlington Heights, IL.

Dietary Supplements for Speed and Power

Hundreds of sport supplements claim they can improve speed and power, but few of those claims are supported by competent science. Athletes should stay focused on what is known to work; nothing beats the right combination of proper training and good nutrition to support the many adaptations to training. A sport nutrition supplement might provide a small additional performance benefit but only if a solid foundation of proper training and food-first nutrition practices are already in place.

Some supplements have been shown to be associated with improved speed and power output, at least in laboratory settings. Creatine and beta-alanine are two examples of dietary supplements that have been shown to increase speed and power under certain circumstances. Creatine supplementation has been shown to improve repeated high-intensity exercise performance, so creatine loading could be a performance aid in training sessions that include repeated explosive movements. Beta-alanine is an amino acid supplement that may increase the ability of muscle cells to buffer lactic acid, helping to sustain high-intensity efforts.

Before recommending a supplement to an athlete or client, you need to consider the risk-to-benefit relationship of supplement use. Is there a demonstrated benefit? If so, what are the related risks to health or competition eligibility due to the possibility of banned substances? These are not easy questions, and it is always best to seek the advice of someone qualified to sort through the science and provide advice. Sport dietitians (Registered Dietitian Nutritionists—RDNs—with training in sport nutrition) can help assess the risk-to-benefit ratio associated with the use of dietary supplements.

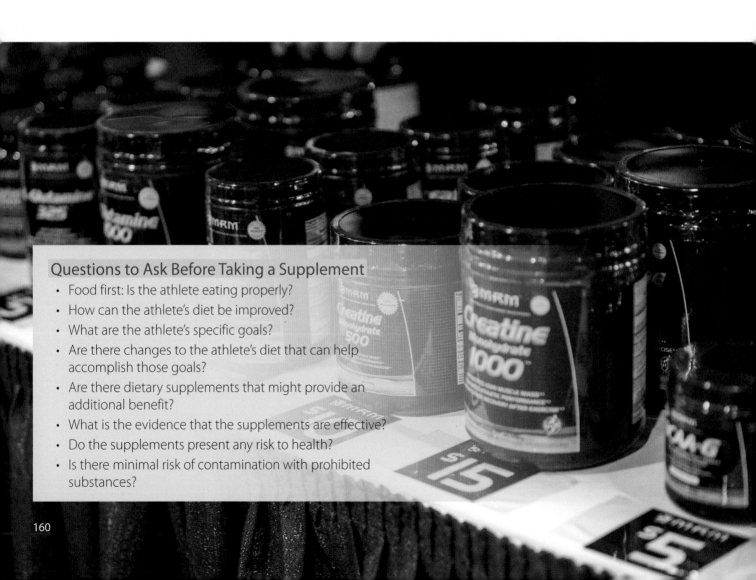

Questions to Ask Before Taking a Supplement

- Food first: Is the athlete eating properly?
- How can the athlete's diet be improved?
- What are the athlete's specific goals?
- Are there changes to the athlete's diet that can help accomplish those goals?
- Are there dietary supplements that might provide an additional benefit?
- What is the evidence that the supplements are effective?
- Do the supplements present any risk to health?
- Is there minimal risk of contamination with prohibited substances?

Chapter Summary

- Speed and power are critical components of all physical activities, including those conducted at low intensities.
- Speed is a measure of the rate of motion and is an important aspect of power—the rate at which energy is transferred.
- The adaptations to speed and power training differ from, but are complementary to, those resulting from endurance training. The opposite is also true.
- HIIT can improve speed and power as well as $\dot{V}O_{2max}$ and endurance performance.
- Plyometric training, ballistic training, interval training, and cross-training can all be part of a program to improve speed and power.

Review Questions

1. Describe the difference between speed and power.
2. Identify three adaptations to speed and power training that contribute to improved performance.
3. Discuss how ballistic training differs from plyometric and eccentric training.
4. Define metabolic flexibility and describe its importance to athletes.
5. Explain the advantages and disadvantages of cross training.

CHAPTER NINE

Training for Aerobic Endurance

Objectives

- Understand the metabolic and physiological underpinnings associated with endurance performance.
- Appreciate how the body responds to prolonged physical activity and adapts to endurance training.
- Learn the importance of the anaerobic threshold to endurance performance.

When you think of aerobic endurance, it's natural to think of marathon running, cross-country skiing, road cycling, open-water swimming, and other sports and activities of long duration. After all, success in those kinds of activities requires a large aerobic capacity; in other words, success in endurance events requires a large maximal oxygen uptake ($\dot{V}O_{2max}$), among other characteristics. Aerobic capacity is just as important in everyday life. Although top endurance athletes have $\dot{V}O_{2max}$ values in excess of 70 ml/kg/min (60 ml/kg/min in women), at the other end of the spectrum are individuals for whom a $\dot{V}O_{2max}$ of just 15 ml/kg/min is needed to accomplish the basic tasks of everyday living. In contrast, sedentary men and women typically have $\dot{V}O_{2max}$ values of 30 to 40 ml/kg/min. Proper training can obviously increase $\dot{V}O_{2max}$, and the extent of that increase depends on a variety of factors, only some of which are under an athlete's or client's control.

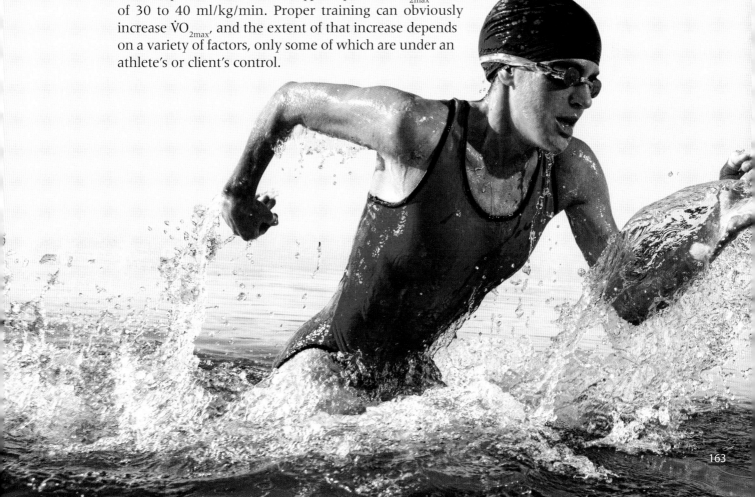

What Are the Main Adaptations to Aerobic Training?

At rest and during exercise, muscles use oxygen to produce much of the ATP required for contracting muscle cells and for fueling other tissues throughout the body. At rest, you breathe slowly but at a rate sufficient to expose your lungs to ample oxygen and flush out the carbon dioxide constantly produced during energy metabolism. Oxygen molecules enter the bloodstream, bind to hemoglobin molecules in red blood cells, and are transported through arteries, arterioles, and capillaries for delivery to individual cells. Once inside cells, the oxygen molecules enter the mitochondria for use in the electron transport chain for the continuous production of ATP. During exercise, all those events accelerate: The rate and depth of breathing increase, the heart beats faster, the left ventricle fills with more blood, cardiac output increases, arterioles dilate, and more muscle capillaries fill with blood. Inside muscle cells, the increased oxygen delivery is matched by increases in the rate of glycogen breakdown, fatty-acid catabolism, glycolysis, lactate production, the Krebs cycle, and the electron transport chain. All those events are reflected by one measurement: $\dot{V}O_{2max}$. The higher the $\dot{V}O_{2max}$, the faster the muscles can produce the ATP required for contraction.

An increase in $\dot{V}O_{2max}$ is one of many adaptations that occur with endurance training. Because it is just one of many adaptations, a high $\dot{V}O_{2max}$ is not necessarily a good predictor of successful endurance performance. For example, there is no doubt that a person with a $\dot{V}O_{2max}$ of 55 ml/kg/min has a competitive advantage over someone with a $\dot{V}O_{2max}$ of 40 ml/kg/min, but the advantage may not hold true when competing against someone with a $\dot{V}O_{2max}$ of 50 ml/kg/min. In essence, $\dot{V}O_{2max}$ is simply a measure of the body's ability to extract oxygen from inhaled air and deliver it into the mitochondria in active muscle cells. There is an upper limit to that ability, and that upper limit is in large part determined by the heart's

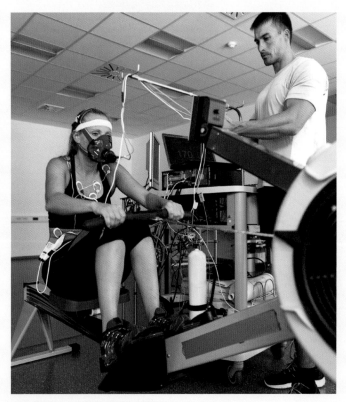

capacity to pump blood, the cardiac output. The upper limit for cardiac output determines the capacity not only for endurance exercise but also for the ability to live independently later in life. Not all people aspire to be endurance athletes, but all people do value the freedom associated with being able to take care of themselves. Proper training can enhance functional capacity, be it to improve physical performance or simply to enhance quality of life.

As mentioned in chapter 3, $\dot{V}O_{2max}$ is the maximal volume of oxygen used by the body during each minute of intense exercise. The formula by which $\dot{V}O_{2max}$ is calculated is simple:

$$\dot{V}O_{2max} = \text{cardiac output} \times \text{a-}\bar{v}O_{2diff}$$

You learned that cardiac output is the product of stroke volume multiplied by heart rate and is expressed in liters per minute; in other words, cardiac output is the volume of blood that the heart pumps out each minute. The $a\text{-}\bar{v}O_{2diff}$ refers to the difference between the amount of oxygen in arterial blood and the amount in venous blood. For example, if arterial blood contains 20 milliliters of oxygen per 100 milliliters of blood while venous blood contains 14 milliliters, the $a\text{-}\bar{v}O_{2diff}$ is 6 milliliters of oxygen per 100 milliliters of blood. This equation is often referred to as the *Fick equation*, named after the scientist who developed it in the 1800s. Fortunately, $\dot{V}O_2$ can be calculated without measuring cardiac output or taking blood samples. Measuring the O_2 and CO_2 contents of inspired and expired air, along with pulmonary ventilation (the volume of air moving through the lungs each minute), enable precise measures of oxygen consumption, even on a breath-by-breath basis.

Obviously, the most important adaptation for athletes is improved performance. Better performance is also an interest of exercise scientists because improving the capacity for exercise is important not only for athletic performance but also because improved aerobic fitness is related to a reduced risk of noncommunicable diseases such as heart disease, obesity, and diabetes; improved recovery from surgery; as well as all the other health-related issues listed in figure 9.1.

> Mitochondria contain more than 1,000 different proteins. Training increases the number of mitochondria, antioxidants within mitochondria, and a variety of proteins that protect the muscle cells against stress.

FIGURE 9.1 Regular exercise and the improved fitness that results help reduce the risk of many diseases and disorders.

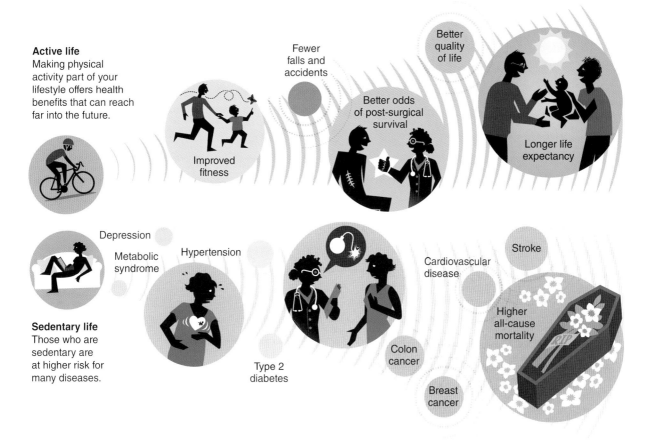

Active life
Making physical activity part of your lifestyle offers health benefits that can reach far into the future.

Improved fitness

Fewer falls and accidents

Better quality of life

Better odds of post-surgical survival

Longer life expectancy

Sedentary life
Those who are sedentary are at higher risk for many diseases.

Depression

Metabolic syndrome

Hypertension

Type 2 diabetes

Colon cancer

Breast cancer

Cardiovascular disease

Stroke

Higher all-cause mortality

Why Is $\dot{V}O_{2max}$ So Important for Endurance?

Aerobic capacity—as measured by $\dot{V}O_{2max}$—reflects the capacity of muscles to produce ATP from the aerobic metabolism of carbohydrate (glucose) and fat (fatty acids). To improve fitness and endurance performance, the ability to produce ATP aerobically—and to sustain that production—has to increase. That ability is reflected in $\dot{V}O_{2max}$.

As mentioned, the athlete with the highest $\dot{V}O_{2max}$ does not always finish first. Many other factors interact to determine overall athletic success; in endurance sports, $\dot{V}O_{2max}$ is just one of those factors. However, it is one of the major factors in the ability to complete endurance events. Figure 9.2 summarizes the main physiological changes that underlie an improvement in $\dot{V}O_{2max}$.

Performance Nutrition Spotlight

To improve endurance performance, the American College of Sports Medicine recommends consuming 30 to 60 grams of carbohydrate per hour during exercise lasting more than one hour (up to 90 g per hr if exercise lasts longer than 2 hr). Mixtures of simple sugars such as sucrose, glucose, and fructose work best at promoting rapid absorption and increasing carbohydrate oxidation in active muscle cells.

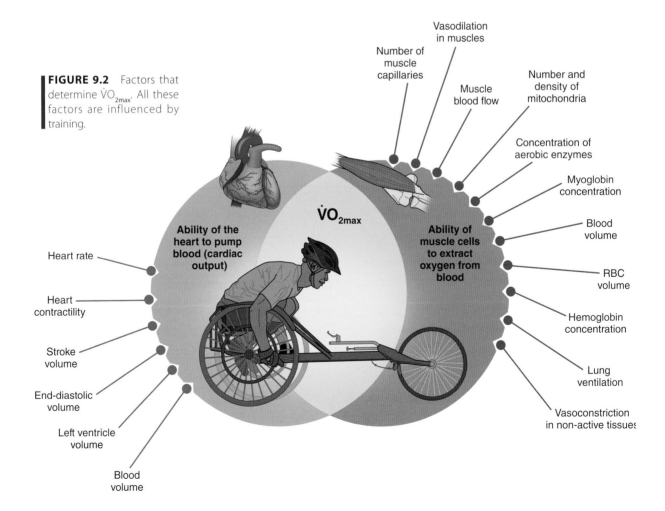

FIGURE 9.2 Factors that determine $\dot{V}O_{2max}$. All these factors are influenced by training.

Some athletes who compete in ultraendurance events that can last 12 hours or more have experimented with high-fat, low-carbohydrate diets (keto diets) in an attempt to maximize fat oxidation, spare muscle glycogen, and improve performance. Such diets require severe restriction of carbohydrate intake (<10% daily calories) and result in ketosis—increased production of ketones such as acetoacetate and beta-hydroxybutyrate from fatty acids. Research has shown that keto diets do increase fat oxidation and spare glycogen. However, overall performance often suffers because the body's metabolic flexibility is hampered. In other words, athletes perform best when training and diet promote maximal metabolic flexibility—the capacity to use both fat and carbohydrate as fuel during exercise.

It is true that during prolonged exercise, muscles naturally produce free radical molecules that can damage important structures and functions inside muscle cells. It is also true that there are antioxidants within cells—molecules such as glutathione, peroxidase, and superoxide dismutase—that protect cells against damage by free radicals. Dietary antioxidants such as vitamins C, E, and beta-carotene (vitamin A) also provide protection. What is not true is that consuming large amounts of these vitamins increases protection from free radicals. Studies show that supplementing with antioxidant vitamins does not enhance performance or aid adaptations to training. In fact, antioxidant supplementation may retard adaptations because some free radical production and temporary inflammation are needed to produce beneficial adaptations. In addition, supplementing with large doses of antioxidants will reduce the natural production of antioxidants in cells. Athletes should be encouraged to eat a varied diet containing fruits and vegetables to provide muscle cells with natural vitamins and phytonutrients that aid in antioxidant protection at little risk of impeding adaptations.

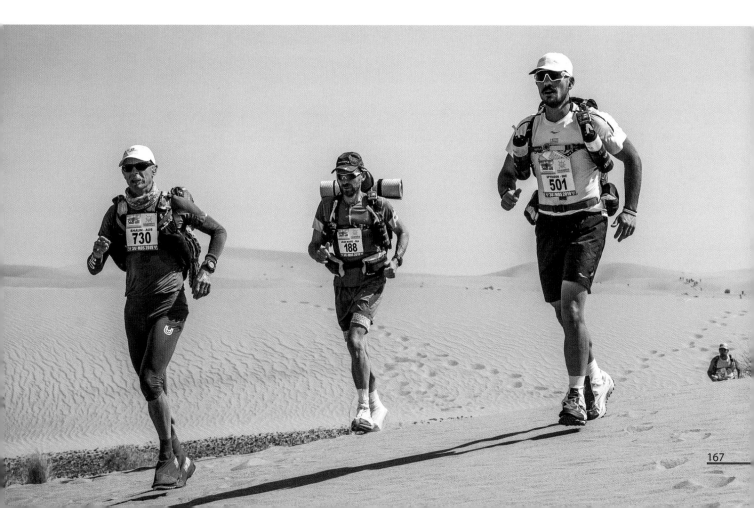

What Factors Determine
How Much Aerobic Capacity Improves?

One obvious answer to this question is training. Adhering to an endurance training program is perhaps the single most important factor that determines how much aerobic capacity ($\dot{V}O_{2max}$) improves. However, individual responses to an aerobic training program vary widely. Following are key factors that combine to determine the overall improvement in $\dot{V}O_{2max}$:

- *Initial fitness.* An athlete whose $\dot{V}O_{2max}$ is high before training will usually have a smaller improvement than an athlete who begins training with a low $\dot{V}O_{2max}$.

- *Heredity.* A person's genetics establishes the upper limit of improvement in $\dot{V}O_{2max}$ as the result of training. (Keep in mind that there is currently no genetic test that can accurately predict athletic potential.) Genetics also determines the extent to which people respond to training. High responders improve more quickly and to a greater extent than low responders.

- *Sex.* $\dot{V}O_{2max}$ in women is typically 10% to 15% lower than that in similarly trained men, although top female athletes often have $\dot{V}O_{2max}$ values that are greater than many male athletes.

- *Training.* Even after $\dot{V}O_{2max}$ plateaus with training, endurance performance can still improve as movement economy and anaerobic threshold continue to increase with training.

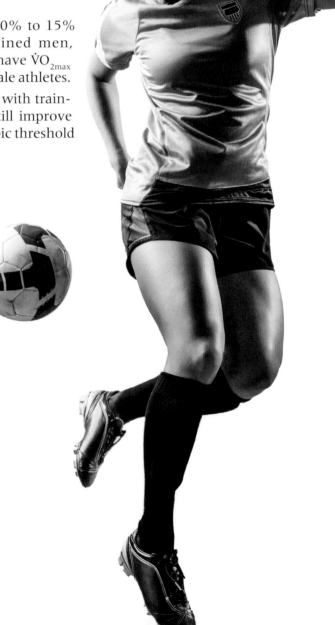

In a muscle, some mitochondria are located just inside the sarcolemma and some are located between the myofibrils. These two types of mitochondria seem to differ in how they respond to training, but both types do improve their capacity to produce ATP.

Ever since the late 1960s, East African runners—from countries such as Ethiopia and Kenya—have been consistently successful in middle- and long-distance running events. Does their heredity—their genetic makeup—give those runners a competitive advantage that other racers cannot hope to achieve? Or do nongenetic factors such as living at altitude or being very active as children interact to produce supremacy in distance running? This puzzle has not yet been solved, but the following are key characteristics that likely combine to help explain the success of East African distance runners.

Heredity: a genetic predisposition for a high aerobic capacity

Physical activity as kids: extensive running, walking, cycling, and overall physical activity throughout childhood

Living and training at altitude: stimulates high hemoglobin, hematocrit, and blood volume

Body size and dimensions: longer legs and a shorter torso favor better running economy

Muscle fiber type: a higher percentage of type I fibers with great oxidative capacity

Traditional diet: carbohydrate-rich diets to help speed recovery and promote adaptations to training

Economic motivation: success at distance running is seen as one way to improve economic and social standing

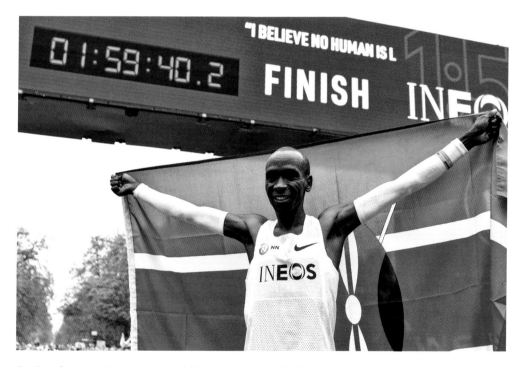

On October 12, 2019, 34-year-old Kenyan runner Eliud Kipchoge finished a staged marathon run in Vienna, Austria, in 1:59:40, breaking the 2-hour barrier for the first time. At that time, Kipchoge was also the official world record holder, having run 2:01:39 in the 2018 Berlin marathon. His Vienna marathon will not count as a world record because it was held on a 6-mile loop with a continuing rotation of pace runners aiding Kipchoge's effort.

Why Is the Anaerobic Threshold Important?

During endurance exercise, blood lactate levels increase from resting values and then remain fairly steady until the push for the finish line. If exercise intensity creeps too high, blood lactate begins to accumulate, indicating that the active muscle cells are relying more and more on glycolysis—anaerobic metabolism—to produce ATP. If exercise intensity is not reduced, the muscle cell environment becomes increasingly acidic, and it becomes tougher to maintain the increased pace; before too long, fatigue sets in and the pace of exercise slows.

Proper training can increase the anaerobic threshold and reduce the accumulation of lactate. That means a faster pace of exercise, even if $\dot{V}O_{2max}$ remains unchanged (see figure 9.3).

• An athlete who can increase his anaerobic threshold from 75% to 85% of $\dot{V}O_{2max}$ can increase running pace even if $\dot{V}O_{2max}$ remains unchanged.

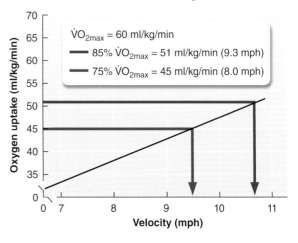

$\dot{V}O_{2max}$ = 60 ml/kg/min
— 85% $\dot{V}O_{2max}$ = 51 ml/kg/min (9.3 mph)
— 75% $\dot{V}O_{2max}$ = 45 ml/kg/min (8.0 mph)

In addition to being a by-product of anaerobic metabolism, lactic acid is also a fuel that heart and skeletal muscles can use to benefit performance.

FIGURE 9.3 Improved anaerobic threshold allows running pace to increase even if $\dot{V}O_{2max}$ does not change. This graph illustrates how an improvement in anaerobic threshold can translate into a much faster race pace.

Based on W.L. Kenney, J.H. Wilmore, and D.L. Costill, *Physiology of Sport and Exercise*, 7th ed. (Champaign, IL: Human Kinetics, 2020), 288.

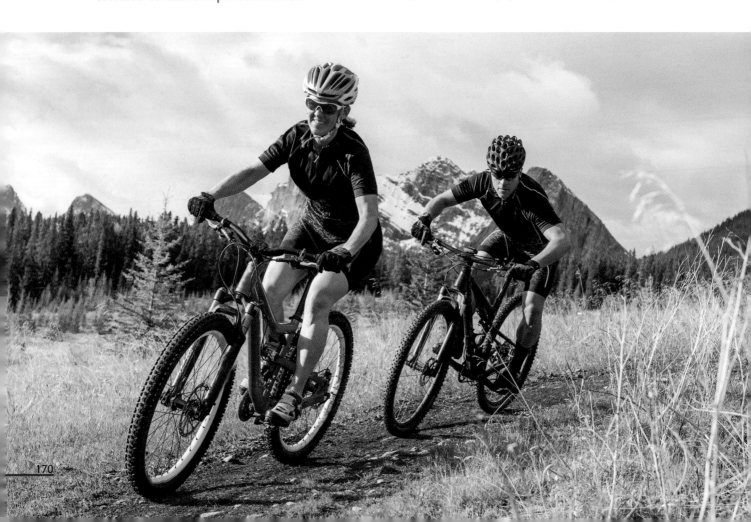

What Other Factors Affect Endurance Performance?

Remember not to confuse aerobic capacity and endurance performance. Although the two are definitely linked—those with greater aerobic capacities tend to have better endurance performance—aerobic capacity eventually plateaus with training, yet endurance performance can continue to improve for years.

One important characteristic in all sports is the energy cost of locomotion, which is referred to as *economy of movement*. Economy of movement is critical for endurance sports because uneconomical movements require ATP energy that does not contribute to forward motion. A simple example of the importance of movement economy is excessive bouncing while running. Each bounce requires energy that is not used for forward progress. Some of that lost energy with each bounce is elastic energy, not ATP energy, but it's also important for athletes to capture the elastic energy in muscles and connective tissues to contribute to forward movement.

Figure 9.4 shows the factors that sport scientists believe are determinants of endurance performance. Training programs for endurance athletes should reflect these characteristics.

Some sport scientists think that in ultraendurance activities such as 100-mile runs, running economy is not as important as other factors—such as lactate threshold—in determining performance.

▌FIGURE 9.4   Determinants of endurance performance.

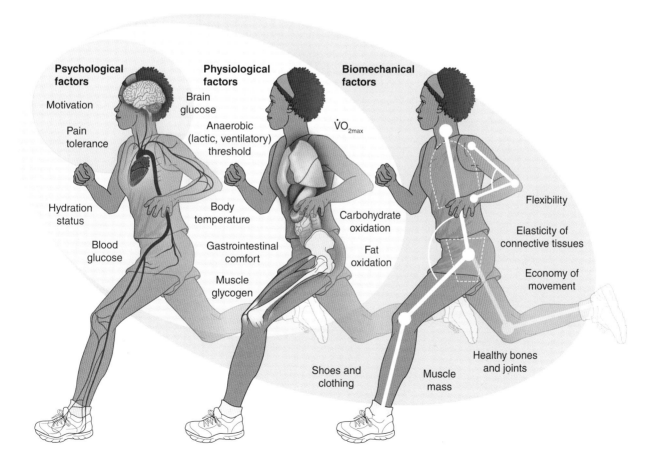

Hematocrit is the scientific name referring to the percentage of blood that is composed of red blood cells. Determining a person's hematocrit is a simple procedure conducted in a laboratory by someone trained and experienced in measuring hematocrit. A small amount of blood is drawn into a thin glass tube and then the tube is spun in a centrifuge to separate the red blood cells from the plasma. Simply measuring the length of the portion composed of the red blood cells and comparing that to the length of the entire content of the tube provide the hematocrit as a percentage of the total.

As with everything in biology, there is no one value that represents normal. In healthy young men, hematocrit is usually about 45%; in other words, 45% of the blood volume is taken up by red blood cells. In healthy young women, the average value is around 40%. (These values apply to people who are at a normal hydration level. Dehydration artificially increases hematocrit because it reduces plasma volume.)

Blood doping and injections of *erythropoietin* (EPO) have been used by some endurance athletes to increase the number of red blood cells, raising the hematocrit and the oxygen-carrying capacity of blood to boost performance. Some athletes do have naturally high hematocrit levels, but most people have lower levels. Normal ranges are 41% to 50% for males and 36% to 44% for females.

Some people mistakenly believe that hematocrit level increases after months of training as the body produces more red blood cells as an adaptation to training. As shown in the illustration, the normal response is for hematocrit to fall slightly with training because even though the body does produce more red blood cells, the increase in plasma volume (the fluid part of the blood) is greater than the increase in red blood cell volume. The blood still carries and delivers more oxygen because there are more red blood cells, more hemoglobin, and a greater blood volume.

Hematocrit levels in excess of 50% increase the risk of heart problems, blood clots, and strokes because blood viscosity rises with hematocrit, making it harder for the heart to pump blood and more likely for clots to occur.

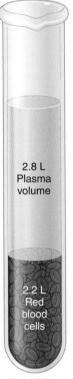

Total blood volume = 5 L
Hematocrit = 44%

2.8 L Plasma volume

2.2 L Red blood cells

Pretraining

Total blood volume = 5.7 L
Hematocrit = 42%

3.3 L Plasma volume

2.4 L Red blood cells

Posttraining

Though training increases both the number of red blood cells and the overall blood volume, posttraining hematocrit is lower because the plasma volume increases more than the volume of red blood cells.

Reprinted by permission from W.L. Kenney, J.H. Wilmore, and D.L. Costill, *Physiology of Sport and Exercise,* 7th ed. (Champaign, IL: Human Kinetics, 2020), 278.

What's the Best Way to Improve Aerobic Endurance?

There is no one best way to improve endurance performance. Endurance athletes across sports have achieved great success using a variety of training approaches. Perhaps the best guidance is that training has to be suited to the physical and psychological characteristics of the athlete and adjusted to where the athlete lives; an endurance athlete who lives in a large city will train differently than if she lived in a hilly rural area. Success is achievable in both scenarios, but the training approach will be different.

Endurance athletes have achieved international and Olympic success by relying on interval training of varying distances, including repeats of 100-meter runs. Long, slow distance training (LSD) has worked for many, as has threshold training designed to improve the anaerobic threshold. Hill training, fartlek training (speed-play training incorporating increased pace at different intervals during a long-duration effort), high-intensity interval training, strength training, and flexibility exercises can all be part of successful endurance training. The same holds true for those uninterested in sport but motivated to improve fitness; all the same training approaches can be used during low-intensity walking, swimming, biking, and other activities.

When designing a training program to improve aerobic capacity and endurance performance, here are some general guidelines that can be manipulated to suit training programs of varying durations and goals:

> Increasing cardiac output, elevating anaerobic threshold, and improving the economy of effort should be the top goals of training programs for endurance athletes.

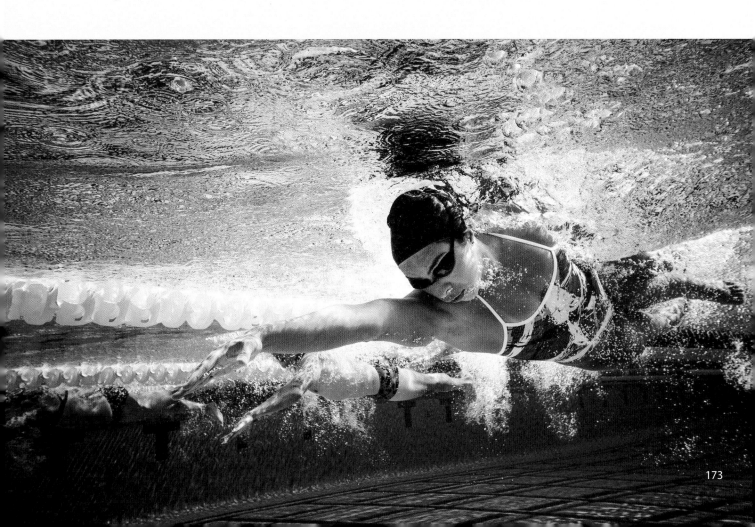

1. *Start out light and fun.* Whether the client is an experienced athlete returning from the off-season or someone new to training, start by developing a solid training base as the foundation for the longer, more demanding training to come. Here are examples:

- Use a strength training circuit with light weights and high reps. Gradually progress over several weeks to heavier weights and fewer reps.
- Use low-intensity, low-mileage walks, runs, rides, and swims focusing on proper mechanics (improved economy of movement), with the occasional hill or similar challenge to begin building stamina. Gradually increase duration and distance over several weeks. Focus less on exercise intensity.
- Begin to acquaint the athlete or client with the demands of high-intensity interval training by using a short session of interval training no more than twice each week. Gradually increase this intensity over weeks.

2. *Gear up for more.* Prepare the athlete for competition. Once a satisfactory training base has been established and the competitive season is approaching, athletes should be physically prepared and mentally motivated to step up training intensity and duration. For clients interested in improved fitness, this phase of training will get them to the next level.

- Change the strength training emphasis to developing sustained muscular power along with the improved core strength required for endurance competition. This is also a time to introduce simple agility exercises that endurance athletes often neglect as well as focus on exercises that develop sport-specific strength.
- Gradually increase the duration and intensity of training, incorporating a mix of anaerobic threshold training, low-intensity and long-duration efforts, speed-play (fartlek) training, and high-intensity interval training (HIIT).
- Increase training intensity and duration gradually, with built-in periods when training load plateaus or even decreases for a few days or a week to allow for recovery and adaptation.
- Continue to emphasize the importance of proper mechanics.

3. *Train during the competitive season.* Once competitions begin (or in the case of the fitness client, once a new level of fitness has been established), the training program should change to reflect the added stress of competition as well as the need for continued improvement while reducing the risks of injury and overtraining.

- Transition strength training from weight and machine resistance training to body-weight exercises and resistance bands to maintain or improve strength gains, with a continued emphasis on sport-specific movements.
- Allow the duration and distance of long efforts to level off. Gradually increase the intensity to reflect the demands of the competitive events.
- Limit high-intensity training to one day per week; other sessions should be devoted to low-intensity recovery training and sessions with limited durations of sustained race-pace training.

4. *Taper for championships.* This period of the training season can differ dramatically depending on the nature of the championship event and the individual

needs of the athletes or clients. Tapering should begin two to four weeks ahead of the final event, customized to the individual's physical and psychological needs for reduced training and rest.

- Transition strength training into a maintenance and injury-prevention program using stability balls, elastic bands, and body-weight exercises.
- In endurance training, maintain aspects of the duration and distance that reflect the championship events. Threshold-intensity training helps sustain the speed required for racing.

With endurance training, the body adapts in incredible ways, as shown in table 9.1.

Endurance training suggestions courtesy of Bill Bishop, Head Coach at Bishop Racing (www.bishop-racing. com), CEO at The Everest Platform, Chicago, IL.

TABLE 9.1 **Adaptations to Endurance Training**

Cardiorespiratory adaptations	Muscle cell adaptations
Resting heart rate decreases about 1 bpm/week. Resting heart rates less than 50 bpm are not unusual in endurance athletes.	Increased ability to extract oxygen from the blood (increased a-$\dot{V}O_{2diff}$).
Heart rates during submaximal exercise are lower but maximal heart rate is unchanged.	Myoglobin content can increase by 80%.
Faster recovery of heart rate after hard efforts.	Increased mitochondrial size and number.
Increased maximal ventilation of the lungs.	Increased content and activity of oxidative enzymes involved in producing ATP.
Increased blood volume.	Increased use of fatty acids during submaximal exercise (reduced RER), reducing reliance on muscle glycogen.
Increased volume of the left ventricle.	Increased cross-sectional area of type I muscle fibers.
Increased left ventricle wall thickness and strength of contraction.	Increased critical power (lactate/anaerobic threshold).
Increased end diastolic volume (improved filling of the heart between beats).	Improved movement economy.
Increased maximal cardiac output (due to increased stroke volume).	
Increased number and density of muscle capillaries.	
Increased capillary recruitment.	
Increased blood flow to muscle cells.	
Improved distribution of blood from inactive tissues to active muscle cells.	
Decreased vascular resistance (makes it easier for the heart to pump blood).	
Increased red blood cell mass.	
Increased hemoglobin content.	
Unchanged or slightly reduced hematocrit.	
Reduced blood viscosity (makes it easier for the heart to pump blood).	
$\dot{V}O_{2max}$ increases by 10%-20%.	

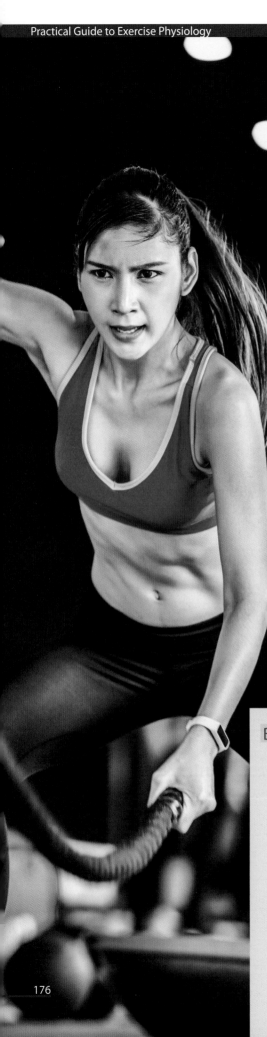

If the benefits of training are specific to the type of training, then the majority of an endurance athlete's training should include activities that stress the aerobic production of ATP from carbohydrate and fat. With that obvious observation in mind, why should endurance athletes spend any time doing anaerobic training? Your common sense has probably already provided an important part of that answer: Endurance athletes need some sprint capacity—some anaerobic capacity—to pass competitors quickly and to sprint to the finish line when needed. But, as the list below illustrates, there are other ways endurance athletes can benefit from anaerobic and high-intensity interval training.

Other variations of high-intensity training can benefit aerobic capacity and performance. Lactate threshold, anaerobic capacity, and even aerobic capacity can be improved by training that integrates repeated high-intensity bouts in an endurance workout. As an example, exercising hard for 3 minutes and then easier for 5 minutes, repeated throughout an hour-long run, cycle, or cross-country ski workout, can improve anaerobic threshold. Endless variations of this kind of speed-play (fartlek) training as well as classic interval training can add variety and high-intensity challenge to endurance workouts.

> HIIT benefits endurance athletes by improving sprint capacity, increasing maximal power output, and providing an additional stimulus for producing the adaptations required for improving aerobic capacity.

Benefits and Characteristics of HIIT for Endurance Athletes

- HIIT increases both aerobic and anaerobic ATP production in muscle cells. HIIT induces increases in $\dot{V}O_{2max}$, blood volume, and oxidative enzymes that are similar to increases seen with conventional endurance training.
- Repeated sprints or high-intensity exercise bouts lasting 20 seconds to 3 minutes, followed by low-intensity activity, improve anaerobic and aerobic capacities.
- Effective HIIT can be accomplished in as little as 20 minutes.
- A small amount of HIIT is as effective as a much larger amount of traditional endurance training at improving the physiological and metabolic capacities that lead to improved endurance performance.
- HIIT should not totally replace conventional aerobic training, but it can be used periodically to give endurance athletes a new challenge that will benefit their performance.

Should Endurance Athletes Engage in Strength Training?

This topic is covered briefly in chapter 8, and it's good news for endurance athletes. The short story is that the benefits of endurance training are not reduced by strength training (but the benefits of strength training can be blunted by too much endurance training). A well-designed strength training program can help endurance athletes maintain or even build muscle mass, an important adaptation during long training seasons.

Although endurance runners and cyclists are often lean, maintaining adequate muscle mass is important for sustaining performance. Loss of muscle mass due to heavy training and inadequate energy (caloric) intake will impair performance. A 30-minute strength training program conducted twice each week can be enough to help prevent the loss of muscle mass.

Open-water swimmers, triathletes, cyclists, and cross-country skiers are good examples of endurance athletes for whom upper- and lower-body musculature is important for success in their sports. Both off-season and in-season strength training are essential for increasing strength and preserving or enhancing muscle mass, adaptations that allow endurance athletes to train and compete at higher levels.

As an example, if a distance swimmer's maximal strength in the latissimus dorsi before a competitive season is 100 pounds (45 kg) and each race requires the swimmer to exert 65 pounds (30 kg) with each arm stroke, the swimmer is repeatedly using 65% of maximal strength. If that swimmer were able to increase maximal strength in the latissimus dorsi to 120 pounds (54 kg), swimming at the same pace would require only 54% of maximal strength, making the effort easier. If the swimmer picked up the pace to use 65% of the new maximal strength, the applied force would be 78 pounds (35 kg), enabling the swimmer to go faster at the same relative effort as before.

Performance Nutrition Spotlight

Training with low muscle glycogen stores has been shown to increase oxidative enzymes involved in carbohydrate and fat oxidation, adaptations that often lead to improved endurance performance. This "train low" strategy should be used only periodically because the capacity for training is dramatically reduced in times of low muscle glycogen. In addition, it is helpful for athletes to increase their protein intake when training with low glycogen to ensure they stay in positive protein balance.

Suggestions for Combining Endurance and Strength Training

- Keep an eye on daily fatigue levels whenever athletes combine intense strength training with demanding endurance training in the same week. Reduce workload if training performance begins to suffer.
- After a hard session of strength training, athletes should ideally have at least 12 hours of recovery before undertaking endurance training.
- Sufficient time is needed after demanding sessions of strength training to allow for recovery of proper running, cycling, or swimming mechanics.
- If possible, plan endurance training before strength training. For example, do endurance training in the morning, with strength training in the afternoon or evening.
- When athletes shift their focus to endurance training, one or two strength workouts per week is enough to maintain muscle strength.
- Vary the mode, duration, and intensity of strength training to optimize adaptations and prevent strength training from interfering with endurance adaptations.

References: Berryman, N. et al. 2018. Strength training for middle- and long-distance performance: a meta-analysis. *Int J Sports Physiol Perform.*13(1):57-63.

Doma, K. et al. 2019. Training considerations for optimising endurance development: an alternate concurrent training perspective. *Sports Med.* 49(5):669-682.

Why Is Endurance Capacity Important for Sprinters and Team-Sport Athletes?

Increased aerobic capacity is the primary defense against fatigue for any athlete or client regardless of sport or activity. Even high-intensity sports stress an athlete's aerobic capacity because recovery from repeated explosive movements relies on aerobic metabolism. And low-intensity sports such as golf and baseball have an important aerobic component because of the long duration of those activities.

Fatigue can hinder performance in all sports. Improved aerobic capacity can delay the onset of fatigue, benefitting performance even in nonendurance sports. Such activities don't primarily rely on aerobic ATP production during competition, but the ability to continue to sustain mental concentration, recover from repeated explosive bouts of exercise, and withstand training and competing in hot environments all benefit from improved aerobic capacity.

That does not mean that a baseball player needs to train like a cross-country runner. But it does mean that a baseball player can benefit from training designed to improve his aerobic capacity. That type of training may not be a large portion of the player's overall training regimen, but it should not be neglected.

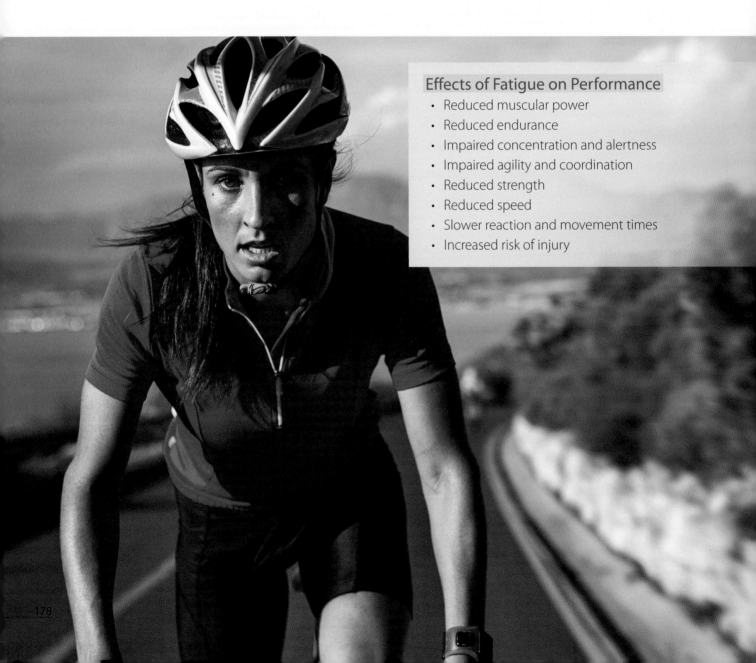

Effects of Fatigue on Performance
- Reduced muscular power
- Reduced endurance
- Impaired concentration and alertness
- Impaired agility and coordination
- Reduced strength
- Reduced speed
- Slower reaction and movement times
- Increased risk of injury

Chapter Summary

- Aerobic training induces numerous adaptations in the muscles, heart, lungs, liver, and other tissues that improve the capacity to exercise longer and harder.
- Improved aerobic fitness is also important for athletes in nonendurance sports because the ability to train and compete in short-duration and stop-and-go sports requires sufficient aerobic fitness to speed recovery and provide the stamina needed for hard training.
- Maximal oxygen consumption ($\dot{V}O_{2max}$) is an important component of aerobic fitness, as is the capacity to sustain a high percentage of $\dot{V}O_{2max}$ and the ability to move economically.
- Genetics plays a role in establishing an upper limit for $\dot{V}O_{2max}$ and in whether people respond quickly or slowly to training.
- The ability to sustain a high percentage of $\dot{V}O_{2max}$ can be measured and expressed in various terms such as the ventilatory threshold, lactate threshold, anaerobic threshold, functional threshold power, or critical power. There are differences among these measures but all refer to the capacity to exercise at a certain percentage of $\dot{V}O_{2max}$, a capacity that can be improved with proper training.
- Periodic HIIT workouts are effective at maintaining or improving $\dot{V}O_{2max}$ and provide a change of pace from endurance training.

Review Questions

1. Explain why the athlete with the highest $\dot{V}O_{2max}$ does not always win endurance competitions.
2. Describe three adaptations to endurance training and explain why each is associated with improved performance.
3. Discuss the importance of the anaerobic threshold to endurance performance.
4. Define hematocrit and explain how it is influenced by training.
5. Describe the benefits of HIIT to endurance adaptations.

PART III

Special Considerations

CHAPTER TEN

Heat, Cold, and Altitude

Objectives

- Learn how training and competing in different environments can present special challenges that make it tougher for the body to perform at its peak.
- Understand how the body responds and adapts to different environments.
- Appreciate the changes in training program design and diet modification required to maximize the body's responses to environmental stress.

Heat, cold, and altitude are among the most common environmental stressors that affect the physiological responses to exercise, altering the body's ability to maintain speed, power, and especially endurance. In simple terms, performance in cool weather is usually better than in cold or hot weather and performance at altitude is impaired in many events, but in some events can be enhanced (e.g., sprinting, jumping, and some throwing events).

In this chapter, environmental stressors are tackled one at a time because that's a good way to illustrate how the body adjusts and adapts in commonsense ways to various environments. While reading this chapter, keep in mind that your DNA has the built-in capacity to create the new proteins needed to ensure survival and successfully adapt to environmental stressors that you do not normally encounter—such as extreme cold, high heat and humidity, and altitudes above 5,000 feet (1,524 m).

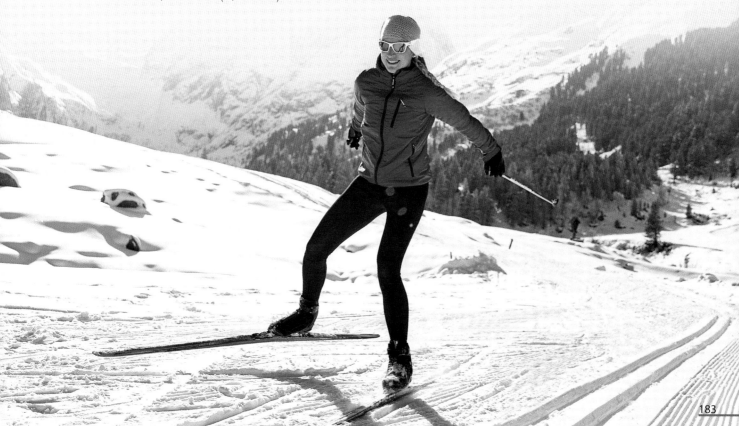

Environmental Heat Impairs Performance

It doesn't have to be very hot for performance to suffer. Research demonstrates that temperatures over 60 °F (15.5 °C) are hot enough to impair performance during prolonged exercise, compared to exercising in temperatures of 40 to 60 °F (4.4-15.5 °C). As the temperature rises above 60 °F, the negative impact on performance becomes progressively greater. Exercising in the heat places an enormous stress on the cardiovascular system; not only is the heart required to pump a lot of blood to active muscles, but it also has to pump a lot of blood to the skin so that the heat produced by contracting muscle cells can be lost to the environment. In addition, the brain is very sensitive to heat, so whenever internal (core) temperature rises substantially, the brain acts to slow down the body—and heat production—to prevent core temperature from rising even further to dangerous levels (an example of "central fatigue").

Figure 10.1 illustrates the fundamental aspects of heat production and loss (heat balance) during exercise. The heat produced by muscles during exercise has to be lost to the environment to prevent overheating. During vigorous exercise, most heat is lost by the *evaporation of sweat* from the skin. On cool days or in cool rooms, you also lose heat by *radiation* as heat moves from your warm body to the cooler surroundings. You can also lose additional heat with the help of *convection*, which is even more effective on windy days or when exercising in front of a fan. *Conduction* is the final avenue for heat loss or gain, but it requires direct contact between the body and a cooler or warmer object. A hockey player lying on an ice rink is one example of conductive heat loss; a child just out of the swimming pool who lies on warm concrete takes advantage of conductive heat gain.

During physical activity, dehydration and hyperthermia are closely linked because fluid is lost from the body during prolonged or intense sweating. Dehydration reduces the heart's ability to supply active muscles with blood and at the same time supply skin with enough blood to aid in heat loss. Staying hydrated during exercise helps protect blood volume and the heart's ability to deliver blood to muscles and skin, preventing or limiting the decline in exercise performance.

From a practical standpoint, for the best performance during hard workouts and competitions, it is always better to be cooler than warmer. Warm-ups should be designed to accomplish just that—warm up the muscles but keep internal temperature from rising too high. Research shows that performance in warm environments is improved by precooling, so some athletes use cold vests and cold-water immersion, rest in air-conditioned spaces, or

> Humans are homeotherms: Core temperature is regulated within a narrow range at rest (36.1-37.8 °C, 97.0-100.0 °F).

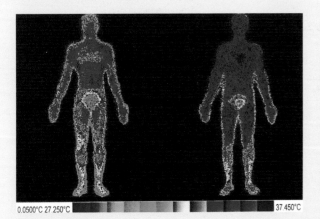 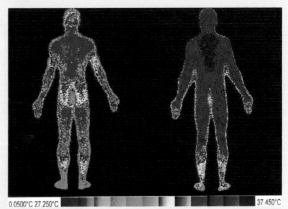

Infrared images showing the heat leaving the (a) front and (b) rear surfaces of the body before and after a run outside in hot, humid weather. In each pair, the pre-run image is shown on the left and the post-run image on the right.

From Department of Health and Human Performance, Auburn University, Alabama. Courtesy of John Eric Smith, Joe Molloy, and David D. Pascoe. By permission of David Pascoe.

consume cold drinks or ice slushies to lower body temperature. Studies also demonstrate that a warm-up lasting 5 to 15 minutes that incorporates a variety of exercise intensities is usually sufficient to cause a small increase in muscle temperature and provide the physical and psychological preparation that most athletes prefer before training and competition. Warming up again after halftime or other breaks in competition can usually be accomplished with 2 minutes of high-intensity movements. Cooling down after exercise in the heat is important if recovery time before the next match is short to ensure that body temperature is lowered as much as possible before beginning again. Sports such as soccer, tennis, volleyball, wrestling, and softball often have tournaments that require athletes to compete multiple times a day for two or more days. Under such conditions, it is critical that athletes cool down and hydrate between competitions.

> Heat stress cannot be measured by temperature alone. Environmental heat stress is determined by a combination of wind speed, relative humidity, radiation, and ambient temperature.

FIGURE 10.1 Body temperature naturally rises during exercise as muscles produce heat. Most of that heat must be lost to the environment to keep internal temperature from climbing dangerously high. Depending on the environmental conditions, heat gain and loss can occur through various channels to ensure the body does not overheat.

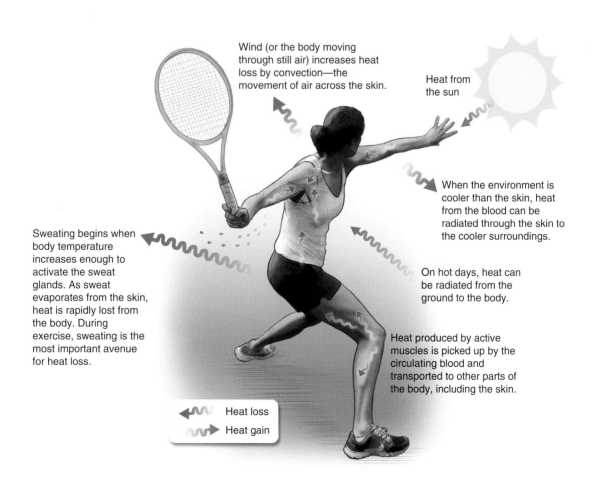

Training in the Heat Improves Performance

How can it be that exercising in the heat impairs performance but training in the heat improves performance? Performance in hot environments is consistently worse than in cooler environments because the body has only so much blood to go around. When blood flow to the skin rises to high levels, as it does during heat exposure and exercise, blood flow to muscles cannot rise high enough to sustain peak performance. But training in the heat—becoming *acclimated* to the heat—improves performance in all environments because of the many adaptations that accompany heat acclimation. Those adaptations are shown in figure 10.2 and are why many elite athletes undergo heat-acclimation training to improve all-weather performance.

Training in the heat benefits performance in cooler environments because the adaptations that occur with heat acclimation—such as increased blood volume—improve the capacity for hard exercise. The benefits of heat acclimation are lost at a rate of about 2.5% for each day without heat exposure, but periodic training sessions in the heat will help maintain those benefits (e.g., training in the heat once every five days).

Full heat acclimation requires training in a warm environment. Just being exposed to heat at rest is not enough. If regular training in hot environments is not possible, the combination of cool weather training plus exposure to passive heat (hot tubs, saunas) may prove beneficial in maintaining heal acclimation.

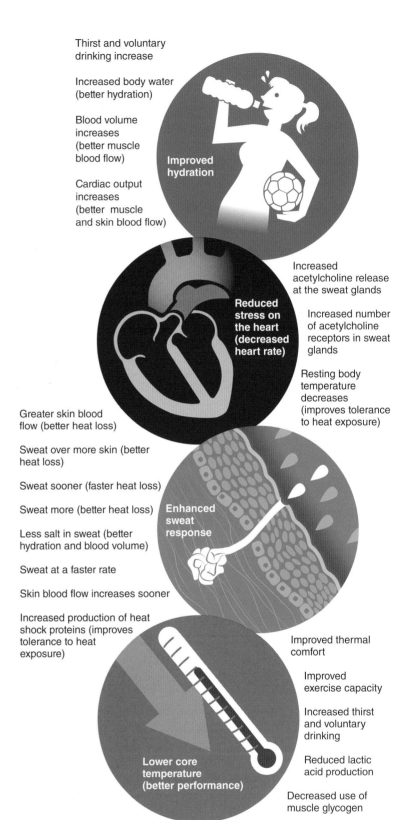

Thirst and voluntary drinking increase

Increased body water (better hydration)

Blood volume increases (better muscle blood flow)

Improved hydration

Cardiac output increases (better muscle and skin blood flow)

Reduced stress on the heart (decreased heart rate)

Increased acetylcholine release at the sweat glands

Increased number of acetylcholine receptors in sweat glands

Resting body temperature decreases (improves tolerance to heat exposure)

Greater skin blood flow (better heat loss)

Sweat over more skin (better heat loss)

Sweat sooner (faster heat loss)

Sweat more (better heat loss)

Enhanced sweat response

Less salt in sweat (better hydration and blood volume)

Sweat at a faster rate

Skin blood flow increases sooner

Increased production of heat shock proteins (improves tolerance to heat exposure)

Improved thermal comfort

Improved exercise capacity

Increased thirst and voluntary drinking

Reduced lactic acid production

Lower core temperature (better performance)

Decreased use of muscle glycogen

FIGURE 10.2 Acclimation to the heat occurs by training in warm weather. Gradually increasing the duration and intensity of workouts over the first two weeks of warm-weather training causes the body to undergo a variety of adaptations that improve the capacity to exercise in the heat. Differences in heat tolerance among people are due to differences in the extent of heat acclimation and fitness level, not to race.

Sweat Is Cool

You know what it's like to sweat, but few understand the true importance of sweating during physical activity or heat exposure. Whenever core body temperature rises above what is called the *sweat threshold*, eccrine sweat glands in the skin begin to produce sweat. You were born with roughly two million sweat glands that enable you to survive hot weather and vigorous physical exercise simply because those glands secrete water onto the surface of the skin. As water molecules evaporate from the skin, heat is lost to the environment. In fact, during intense exercise, 80% of the heat produced by muscles is lost from the body by the evaporation of sweat. Sweat that drips off the skin, however, provides no cooling; it must evaporate.

Sweating does for humans what panting does for dogs, but sweating does it better. Sweating is an effective way to stay safely cool in hot environments. That simple fact explains why humans are better than most animals at being physically active in the heat for prolonged periods. Animals that do not sweat cannot pant fast enough to keep up with the heat production of exercise. In humans, when body temperature increases slightly above normal resting temperature (98.6 °F or 37 °C), the hypothalamus in the brain senses the increase in temperature and signals the sympathetic nervous system to dilate blood vessels in the skin and activate sweat glands. (See figure 10.3.)

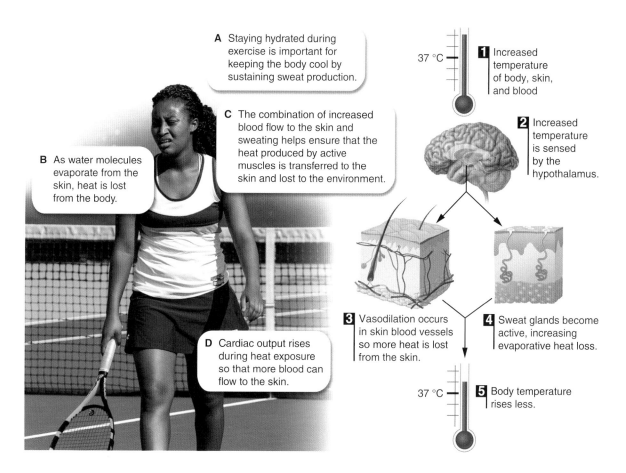

A Staying hydrated during exercise is important for keeping the body cool by sustaining sweat production.

C The combination of increased blood flow to the skin and sweating helps ensure that the heat produced by active muscles is transferred to the skin and lost to the environment.

B As water molecules evaporate from the skin, heat is lost from the body.

D Cardiac output rises during heat exposure so that more blood can flow to the skin.

37 °C

1 Increased temperature of body, skin, and blood

2 Increased temperature is sensed by the hypothalamus.

3 Vasodilation occurs in skin blood vessels so more heat is lost from the skin.

4 Sweat glands become active, increasing evaporative heat loss.

37 °C

5 Body temperature rises less.

FIGURE 10.3 Sweating is a critical part of temperature regulation because sweating during exercise is the primary way in which humans lose heat to the environment and maintain a safe internal body temperature.

You know how uncomfortable you feel on a hot, humid day. The humidity of the air influences the rate of heat loss because humidity directly affects the evaporation of sweat. When there is more water vapor in the air than on the skin (as usually occurs at very high relative humidities), sweat cannot evaporate from the skin; it literally has no place to go because the surrounding air already contains as much water vapor as it can hold. At the other end of the humidity spectrum, when exercise takes place in a dry, desert environment, sweat can evaporate so quickly from the skin that you hardly notice you're sweating. That rapid evaporation makes for effective heat loss but increases the risk of dehydration because you miss the sweaty skin and clothing that cue you that you're losing fluid and should drink to replace it. As humidity climbs, heat loss is made progressively more difficult, increasing the risk of early fatigue, heat exhaustion, and heatstroke.

Dangers of Exercise in the Heat

There is a limit to the body's ability to lose heat to the environment. When that limit is reached, core temperature will continue to climb if exercise continues. The brain can tolerate internal temperatures of 40 to 41 °C (104-106 °F) for only short periods. The rate at which core temperature increases and the extent to which it rises depends on the intensity and duration of exercise and the environmental conditions. Intense exercise in a hot, humid environment can cause core temperature to quickly climb to dangerous levels. In fact, if heat loss is impeded (as in the dangerous and

Individual sweating rates during the same activity vary widely from person to person, ranging from as little as 300 milliliters (10 oz) per hour to over 3,000 milliliters (100 oz) per hour.

Performance Nutrition Spotlight

During exercise in the heat, pouring cold water on the scalp, face, and neck feels great and provides relief in the form of improved thermal comfort. Unfortunately, that relief is only temporary because the local cooling that occurs is not enough to lower body core temperature. Drinking cool fluids in volumes sufficient to keep dehydration at a minimum is the best way to prevent overheating. Athletes should be encouraged and trained to become better drinkers during exercise so they are able to consume larger volumes more frequently whenever sweat losses are large.

unwise wearing of rubberized clothing during exercise), body temperature can increase into the danger zone in just 15 to 20 minutes at a running pace of only 10 minutes per mile. If core temperature remains at that high level for even a few minutes, *heatstroke* can result. Heatstroke is often fatal because being too hot for too long impairs brain function and causes proteins throughout the body to unravel. The result can be organ system failure and death.

Heat cramps and heat exhaustion are other forms of heat illness but are not life threatening. *Heat cramps* can result from the combination of intense exercise and dehydration. In some athletes, large sodium losses in sweat can cause severe, whole-body muscle cramps. *Heat exhaustion*—unusual fatigue while exercising in the heat—occurs when cardiac output is not able to keep up with the demands of exercise. This occurs when heat gain overwhelms the system and is made significantly worse by dehydration. In normal situations of exercise in the heat, cooling the athlete with fans or air-conditioning, removing excess clothing and headgear, and restoring hydration is usually sufficient to allow core temperature to return to normal before the athlete returns to play. However, heat stroke is a life-threatening emergency that requires that the athlete be cooled as quickly as possible.

Compensable heat stress is when core temperature rises but stabilizes. Noncompensable heat stress is when core temperature continues to rise as the body is unable to lose heat fast enough.

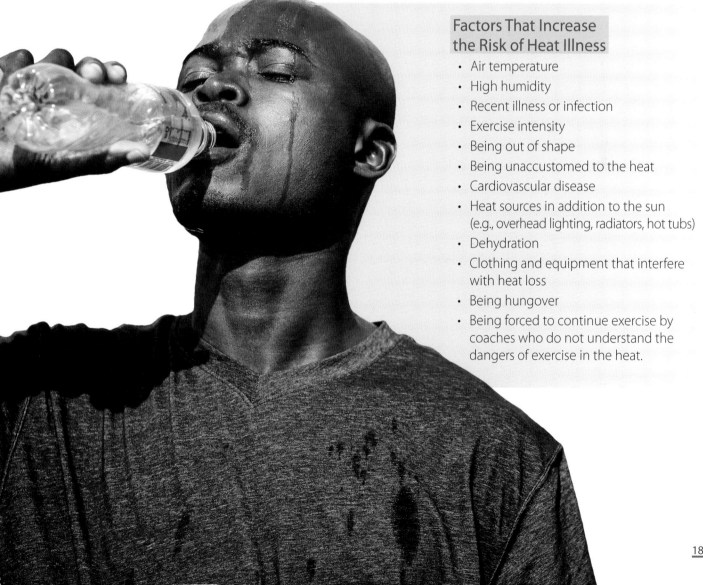

Factors That Increase the Risk of Heat Illness

- Air temperature
- High humidity
- Recent illness or infection
- Exercise intensity
- Being out of shape
- Being unaccustomed to the heat
- Cardiovascular disease
- Heat sources in addition to the sun (e.g., overhead lighting, radiators, hot tubs)
- Dehydration
- Clothing and equipment that interfere with heat loss
- Being hungover
- Being forced to continue exercise by coaches who do not understand the dangers of exercise in the heat.

Heatstroke is characterized by central nervous system dysfunction (confusion, collapse, and sometimes unconsciousness) and is a medical emergency that must be dealt with quickly. Other symptoms of heatstroke can include a core temperature of over 104 °F (40 °C), increased heart rate, decreased blood pressure, and rapid breathing. Cooling the athlete immediately saves lives. While emergency help is on the way, the athlete's torso should be submerged in an ice-water bath to quickly reduce core temperature. If an ice bath is not available, continuous cooling with cold water and wet towels should be used. Athletes who have experienced heatstroke should return to play gradually over a period of weeks while following a heat-acclimation program to ensure that the athlete can tolerate training without signs of central nervous system dysfunction.

Most of the deaths that occur during sudden heat waves are in older individuals who have compromised heart and blood vessel function due to cardiovascular diseases. These individuals may or may not be dehydrated, but often live without air conditioning or fans, and lack the physiological capacity to lose heat fast enough to prevent fatal overheating.

Hot Yoga: Help or Hype?

Hot yoga (Bikram yoga) is a form of yoga exercise consisting of 26 yoga postures during 90-minute sessions in an environment maintained at approximately 104 °F (40 °C) and 40% relative humidity. Truly a hot and sweaty environment! What benefits can be expected from hot yoga? Answering that question requires some reading to identify the benefits that are claimed for hot yoga and the evidence in support of those claims.

In the past, adherents to hot yoga claimed that heavy sweating helped flush toxins from the skin and that the heat allows the body to be more flexible. There is not a lot of scientific research on hot yoga, although a few studies have been conducted. The results of the research confirm what you might expect: Yoga exercise is associated with a modest increase in oxygen consumption ($\dot{V}O_2$) and therefore energy expenditure. Novice yoga students tend to expend less energy than experienced students—a range of approximately 200 to 500 kilocalories (Calories) per 90-minute session. That amounts to roughly 2 to 6 kilocalories per minute, qualifying as light-to-moderate exercise.

Not surprisingly, practicing yoga in the heat raises core temperature and heart rate and provokes sweating. In fact, one study noted that heart rates averaged 72% to 86% of HR_{max}, and novice students had lower values. Heat stress under any circumstance increases strain on the cardiovascular system because of the increase in blood flow to the skin and the loss of body water through sweat. Preventing dehydration by drinking adequate volumes of fluid is essential for protecting cardiovascular health and keeping core temperature from rising to dangerous levels. In addition, exposure to hot environments is contraindicated for those who have multiple sclerosis or cardiovascular disease.

Although there is no reliable evidence that exercise in the heat "softens" the body or that sweat flushes out toxins or impurities, practitioners of hot yoga will experience the physiological benefits of heat acclimation along with the modest improvements in strength, flexibility, and aerobic fitness associated with light-to-moderate exercise.

Pate, J.L., & Buono, M.J. (2014). The physiological responses to Bikram yoga in novice and experienced practitioners. *Alternative Therapies in Health and Medicine, 20*(4):12-18.

Cold Stress Chills Performance

Many environmental conditions can cause the body to lose heat rapidly and reduce core temperature. Fortunately, although cold-weather sports such as ice hockey, downhill skiing, cross-country skiing, and football often take place in frigid conditions, physical activity produces heat and athletes remain warm, especially if their clothing has enough insulation to lessen heat loss. Figure 10.4 illustrates the primary physiological responses to cold exposure.

The effects of acclimation to the cold are less pronounced than those of acclimation to heat. However, athletes who train in the cold can become habituated to the cold, allowing their core temperature to drop slightly without causing shivering. People who are repeatedly exposed to the cold acclimate by increasing metabolic heat production (referred to as *nonshivering thermogenesis*), shivering more, and vasoconstricting blood vessels more effectively. Behavioral adjustments are an important part of temperature regulation in the cold, even more so than in the heat. Adding clothing, moving to a warmer spot, seeking shelter, and adjusting exercise intensity are common behavior adjustments to stay warm.

Sweating during exercise in the cold can speed heat loss if the sweat soaks through clothing.

FIGURE 10.4   During exercise in the cold, the inside of an athlete's clothing can be a very warm place, so skin blood vessels dilate and sweating occurs. But when exercise stops or is reduced to a low intensity, core temperature can quickly fall below normal. When that occurs, the hypothalamus signals the sympathetic nervous system to constrict skin blood vessels (vasoconstrict) and to cause muscles to shiver. Those responses reduce heat loss and increase heat production.

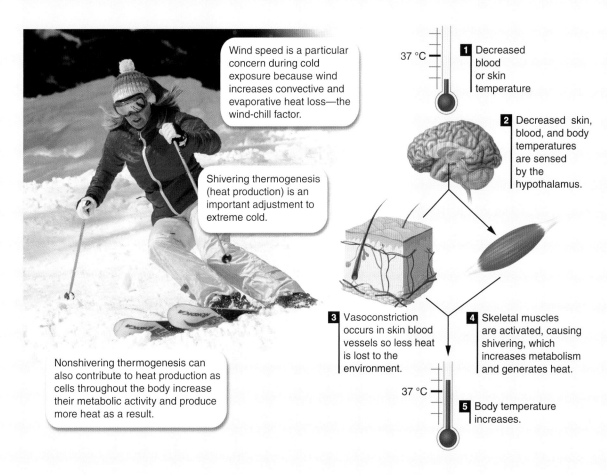

Wind speed is a particular concern during cold exposure because wind increases convective and evaporative heat loss—the wind-chill factor.

Shivering thermogenesis (heat production) is an important adjustment to extreme cold.

Nonshivering thermogenesis can also contribute to heat production as cells throughout the body increase their metabolic activity and produce more heat as a result.

37 °C

1 Decreased blood or skin temperature

2 Decreased skin, blood, and body temperatures are sensed by the hypothalamus.

3 Vasoconstriction occurs in skin blood vessels so less heat is lost to the environment.

4 Skeletal muscles are activated, causing shivering, which increases metabolism and generates heat.

37 °C

5 Body temperature increases.

Exposure to extreme or prolonged cold can overwhelm the body's attempts to maintain temperature. Whenever core temperature drops below normal, fewer motor units in muscle are recruited and the speed at which muscle cells shorten is reduced. Those two changes lessen power production, performance, and heat production. Shivering is an effective way for muscles to produce extra heat, but shivering requires a lot of ATP, which means that muscle glycogen stores can fall quickly. A normal response to exercise and to cold exposure is an increase in catecholamine hormone secretion. Epinephrine (adrenaline) and norepinephrine aid vasoconstriction and increase the release of free fatty acids from fat cells to help fuel shivering muscle cells. In very cold conditions, the vasoconstriction in fat cells actually reduces the release of fatty acids into the bloodstream, thereby reducing some of the fuel that muscle cells need for shivering.

Cold-water exposure is particularly dangerous to the body's ability to maintain temperature. In fact, heat loss in cold water is four times greater than in cold air, even when the body tries to slow heat loss by maximally constricting skin blood vessels and increasing heat production through muscle contractions, increased metabolism, and shivering. As most people know from personal experience, being immersed in or sprayed with cold water can cause body temperature to drop quickly. Water has 26 times greater thermal conductivity than air, which means that being immersed in water rapidly accelerates heat loss from the body. Water that is flowing increases heat loss even further by way of convective cooling.

When core temperature drops below 94 °F (34.5 °C), *hypothermia* sets in and the hypothalamus is not able to control temperature regulation and core temperature continues to drop. The colder the body becomes, the less able the hypothalamus is to control vasoconstriction and increase shivering. Heart rate slows, body temperature drops, drowsiness sets in, and with time coma and death become more likely.

> Adapting to the cold involves cold habituation, metabolic acclimation, and insulative acclimation. It's no accident that cold-water swimmers carry extra body fat!

Performance Nutrition Spotlight

Staying well hydrated during exercise is critical for maintaining important physiological functions and preventing a drop-off in performance. Sweating rate increases in warm environments, so drinking also has to increase to minimize the negative effects of dehydration.

Exercise at Altitude

Chapter 3 discussed the fact that the air you breathe is about 21% oxygen (actually 20.93%) and the rest is nitrogen, aside from a small amount of carbon dioxide. At sea level and low altitudes (lower than 1,500 ft, or 500 m), the atmospheric pressure is high enough to ensure that your lungs are exposed to enough oxygen (O_2) molecules that breathing is easy, especially at rest. But on the highest place on Earth, Mt. Everest, the atmospheric pressure is only 33% of that at sea level. As a result, the O_2 molecules are spread so far apart that breathing becomes difficult because the oxygen content of blood is reduced. (Reduced atmospheric pressure is often referred to as *hypobaria* and reduced oxygen content in blood is called *hypoxia*.) Even though the air at the peak of Mt. Everest still contains 21% oxygen, the atmospheric pressure at 29,028 feet is very low because there is much less air above to create pressure (see figure 10.5.) At sea level, there is a 24-mile-high column of air pressing down on you. On Mt. Everest, that column of air is less than 19 miles high. At altitude, breathing has to be very rapid to introduce enough oxygen into the lungs to satisfy even the low metabolic needs at rest.

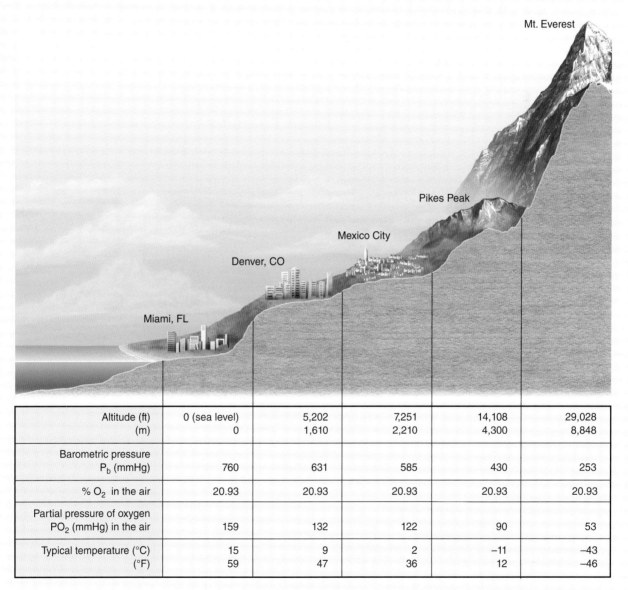

	Miami, FL	Denver, CO	Mexico City	Pikes Peak	Mt. Everest
Altitude (ft)	0 (sea level)	5,202	7,251	14,108	29,028
(m)	0	1,610	2,210	4,300	8,848
Barometric pressure P_b (mmHg)	760	631	585	430	253
% O_2 in the air	20.93	20.93	20.93	20.93	20.93
Partial pressure of oxygen PO_2 (mmHg) in the air	159	132	122	90	53
Typical temperature (°C)	15	9	2	−11	−43
(°F)	59	47	36	12	−46

FIGURE 10.5 As altitude increases, the percentage of oxygen in the air remains the same but the barometric pressure falls, which reduces the partial pressure of oxygen to which lungs are exposed.

Reprinted by permission from W.L. Kenney, J.H. Wilmore, and D.L. Costill, *Physiology of Sport and Exercise,* 7th ed. (Champaign, IL: Human Kinetics, 2020), 333.

Exercise at altitude reduces performance capacity in events lasting more than 2 minutes because maximal aerobic capacity and power are reduced as the result of lower partial pressure of oxygen. This is especially true early after ascent to altitude before adaptations take place. In addition, being at altitude increases the risk of illness, persistent fatigue, weight loss, and overtraining. For purposes of describing the effects of altitude on the human body, elevations are categorized in this way:

Low altitude is 1,500 to 7,000 feet (500-2,000 m) above sea level.

Moderate altitude is 7,000 to 10,000 feet (2,000-3,000 m).

High altitude is 10,000 to 18,000 feet (3,000 to 5,500 m).

Extremely high altitude is more than 18,000 feet (>5,500 m).

Impaired performance can occur above 5,000 feet (1,500 m). In addition to the direct effects of lower atmospheric pressure, colder and drier air at elevation also take a toll. On average, air temperature drops by 1 °C with every 500 feet of elevation. And cold air is dry air, which increases respiratory fluid loss, contributing to dehydration. Figure 10.6 details the physiological adjustments that occur with acute altitude exposure, and table 10.1 shows the height of some of the world's high-altitude cities.

FIGURE 10.6 On first exposure to altitude, several physiological adjustments occur to help in coping with the reduced partial pressure of oxygen in the air.

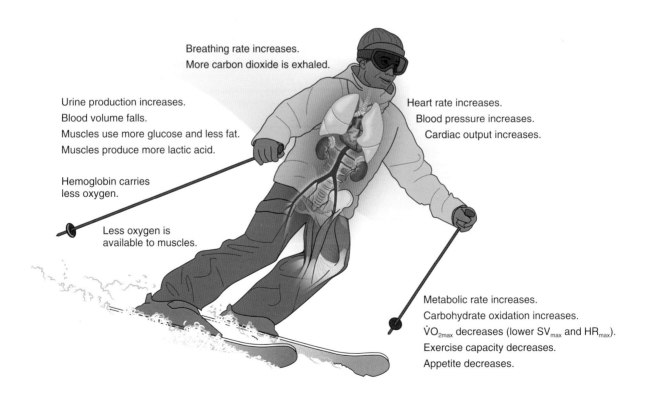

Breathing rate increases.
More carbon dioxide is exhaled.

Urine production increases.
Blood volume falls.
Muscles use more glucose and less fat.
Muscles produce more lactic acid.

Hemoglobin carries less oxygen.

Less oxygen is available to muscles.

Heart rate increases.
Blood pressure increases.
Cardiac output increases.

Metabolic rate increases.
Carbohydrate oxidation increases.
$\dot{V}O_{2max}$ decreases (lower SV_{max} and HR_{max}).
Exercise capacity decreases.
Appetite decreases.

After living at altitude for three weeks or more, a variety of physiological adaptations occur that improve ability to cope with the stress of altitude (see figure 10.7.) The ability to train and compete at altitude improves after living at altitude, but those capacities remain reduced compared to living at sea level.

TABLE 10.1 **Altitudes of Some of the World's Highest Cities**

City	Altitude in feet (meters)
La Rinconada, Peru	16,830 (5,130)
Nagqu, China	14,800 (4,511)
El Alto, Bolivia	13,620 (4,151)
Juliaca, Peru	12,546 (3,824)
Lhasa, Tibet	12,001 (3,658)
La Paz, Bolivia	11,980 (3,652)
Leadville, CO	10,152 (3,094)
Breckenridge, CO	9,602 (2,927)
Divide, CO	9,165 (2,794)
Mammoth Lakes, CA	7,920 (2,414)
Aspen, CO	7,907 (2,410)
Mexico City, Mexico	7,382 (2,250)
Los Alamos, NM	7,320 (2,231)
Laramie, WY	7,163 (2,183)
Summit, VT	7,000 (2,134)
Albuquerque, NM	6,120 (1,865)
Denver, CO	5,202 (1,610)

FIGURE 10.7 After living at altitude for three weeks or more, physiological adaptations occur that improve exercise capacity at altitude but not necessarily at sea level.

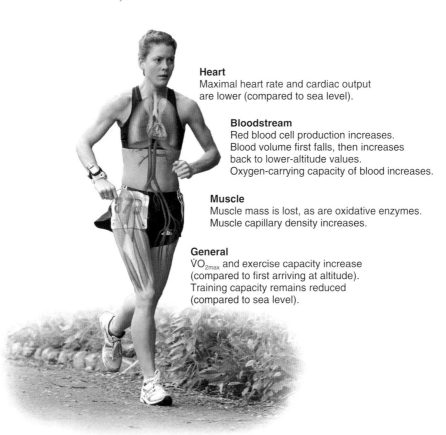

Heart
Maximal heart rate and cardiac output are lower (compared to sea level).

Bloodstream
Red blood cell production increases.
Blood volume first falls, then increases back to lower-altitude values.
Oxygen-carrying capacity of blood increases.

Muscle
Muscle mass is lost, as are oxidative enzymes.
Muscle capillary density increases.

General
$\dot{V}O_{2max}$ and exercise capacity increase (compared to first arriving at altitude).
Training capacity remains reduced (compared to sea level).

Does Training at Altitude Improve Performance at Sea Level?

In many athletes, at least three weeks of living at moderate altitude (7,000-10,000 ft, or 2,000-3,000 m) are needed for respiratory, cardiovascular, and muscle adaptations to occur that allow for harder training. At higher altitudes, more time is often needed. Those various adaptations improve the capacity for aerobic exercise at altitude. But do those adaptations help improve performance at sea level? The answer is still not entirely clear.

The likely reason that altitude training does not consistently improve performance at sea level is that training intensity and duration at altitude is reduced in most athletes; a reduced training stimulus at altitude results in a reduced training response. It appears that most athletes are better off training harder at lower altitudes and benefiting from the increased training stimulus. In addition, spending time at altitude can lead to dehydration and loss of blood volume and muscle mass, all of which impair performance. Also, the additional red blood cells acquired at altitude are destroyed by the body after a week or two at sea level.

Strategies for using altitude exposure as a way to improve performance both at altitude and closer to sea level depend on how much time the athlete can spend at altitude and whether the goal is to prepare for a competition at altitude or to use altitude-related adaptations to gain a competitive edge at sea level. Some coaches and athletes have reported successful performances when competitions occur a few days after returning from altitude training, before some of the altitude-induced training adaptations begin to deteriorate.

For a competition at altitude, athletes should arrive as close as possible to the start of the event so that there is not enough time for the adverse effects of altitude to occur. This option is best when competition is limited to one day. For competitions that are spread over a few days, the best strategy is to train at altitude for at least two weeks before the event so that adverse effects will have come and gone before competition. This approach is best suited for multiday events at altitude.

Perhaps the best approach for endurance athletes is to live at altitude to benefit from the adaptations stimulated by *hypoxia* but train at lower altitudes to maintain a high training stimulus and promote even greater adaptations. In short, *live-high, train-low* seems to make the most theoretical sense, although there is not yet enough research to reach a definitive conclusion for all occasions or all sports. Some athletes use hypoxic sleeping tents to simulate living at altitude to provoke increases in blood volume and hemoglobin that can benefit endurance performance. Research shows that living at 6,600 to 8,200 feet (2,000-2,500 m) seems to provoke the optimal responses. As with all training responses, there is wide variability in how individual athletes respond to altitude exposure. Some athletes will undoubtedly adapt quickly to altitude training and experience performance benefits, while others will struggle with training at altitude and performance will suffer.

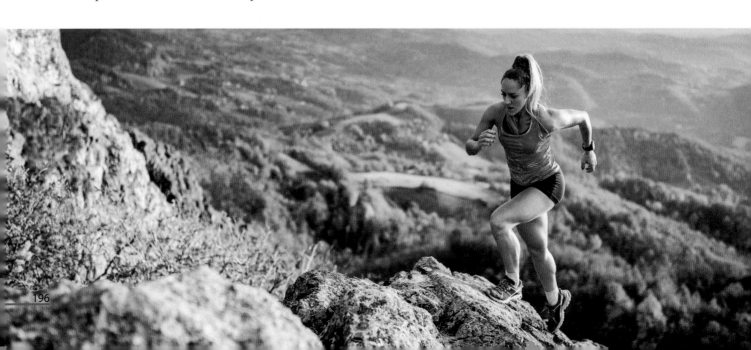

Health Risks at Altitude

As many recreational skiers have experienced, taking a vacation at altitude can sometimes be a real headache. In fact, headaches are the most common symptom of altitude sickness, also known as *acute mountain sickness*. Six hours or more after arriving at altitude, headache, nausea, rapid breathing, and disturbed sleep can occur. After three or four days, the symptoms lessen or disappear. Higher altitudes provoke greater symptoms and in more people. In severe cases, physicians can prescribe medications such as acetazolamide and ibuprofen to ease the symptoms. The responses to altitude vary widely among people and depend on fitness level, nutrition, recovery capacity, sensitivity to hypoxia, and previous exposures to altitude.

While acute mountain sickness can knock vacationers off their skis for a few days, at higher altitudes *high-altitude pulmonary edema* (HAPE) and *high-altitude cerebral edema* (HACE) can be life threatening, as shown in figure 10.8.

Performance Nutrition Spotlight

Living and exercising in environmental extremes require an emphasis on proper nutrition. Exposure to heat, cold, and altitude increases your body's needs for fluid, sodium, carbohydrate, and energy (calories). Increased iron intake (100-200 mg/day) can also be important in helping acclimate to altitude to keep pace with the increased production of hemoglobin and red blood cells.

FIGURE 10.8 High-altitude sickness must be treated immediately.

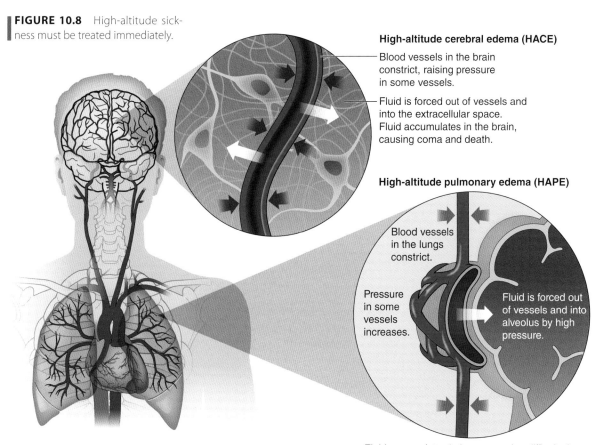

High-altitude cerebral edema (HACE)

Blood vessels in the brain constrict, raising pressure in some vessels.

Fluid is forced out of vessels and into the extracellular space. Fluid accumulates in the brain, causing coma and death.

High-altitude pulmonary edema (HAPE)

Blood vessels in the lungs constrict.

Pressure in some vessels increases.

Fluid is forced out of vessels and into alveolus by high pressure.

Fluid accumulates in lungs, causing difficulty in breathing and increased risk of clotting.

Chapter Summary

- Exercise in warm and humid environments increases the risk of heat-related illnesses because the body is unable to lose heat rapidly enough to prevent a progressive rise in core body temperature.
- Dehydration increases the risk of heat-related illnesses by reducing blood volume and skin blood flow, further impeding heat loss from the body.
- Over a period of 10 days to 2 weeks of daily exercise in the heat, numerous physiological adaptations occur that acclimate the body, allowing for improved exercise capacity and a reduced risk of heat-related illnesses.
- The evaporation of sweat from the skin is the primary avenue for heat loss during exercise.
- Heat exhaustion is an indication of cardiovascular insufficiency, while heatstroke is an indication of central nervous system dysfunction.
- Regular exposure to cold environments results in increased tolerance to the cold as the body makes adjustments in order to reduce heat loss and increase heat production.
- Exercise performance is impaired at altitudes above 5,000 feet (1,500 m) because $\dot{V}O_{2max}$ is reduced due to the lower partial pressure of oxygen.
- Training at altitude induces adaptations in the cardiovascular system that help improve performance at altitude.
- For some athletes, training at altitude improves performance at lower altitudes, but the reduced training load at altitude prevents other athletes from experiencing similar improvements.
- Acute mountain sickness, high-altitude pulmonary edema, and high-altitude cerebral edema are health risks encountered at altitude.

Review Questions

1. List three adaptations that occur with heat acclimation and explain the importance of each.
2. Discuss the primary differences between heat exhaustion and heatstroke.
3. Explain why athletes should consider increasing their daily iron intake when training at altitude.
4. Describe the differences among acute mountain sickness, high-altitude pulmonary edema, and high-altitude cerebral edema.
5. Identify two responses to cold exposure that help stabilize core temperature.

CHAPTER ELEVEN

Training Children and Pregnant Women

Objectives

- Learn how the stage of maturation in children and adolescents and the stage of pregnancy in women influence the design of training programs.
- Discover how children and adolescents respond and adapt to physical activity and regular training.
- Appreciate the factors that should be considered when designing training programs for children, adolescents, and pregnant women.

Athletes and fitness clients come in all shapes, sizes, ages, and physical capacities, each with unique goals, interests, schedules, and challenges. Children and pregnant women represent two categories of athletes and clients who present unique challenges for the design and implementation of effective training programs. Fortunately, regular physical activity positively affects the health of the pregnant woman and her baby and plays an essential role in healthy growth and development during childhood and adolescence.

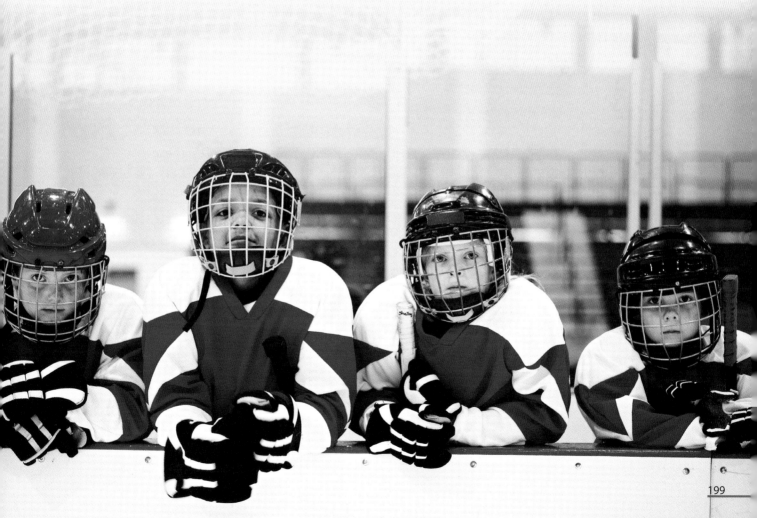

Do Children Respond Differently to Exercise Training?

Regular physical activity has lifelong benefits, regardless of a person's age. That is one of the reasons that children and adolescents are encouraged to get at least 60 minutes of moderate-to-vigorous physical activity each day. The human body is designed for movement, accomplishing physical tasks, and adapting to increased physical demands. You know that lack of physical activity at any time of life has serious negative implications for health, longevity, and quality of life. Sitting for hours at a desk or in front of a television or computer is associated with negative health outcomes that can be minimized simply by moving more often during each day. You also recognize that developing good physical activity habits early in life helps you sustain those habits as you age, especially during the challenging times of life when it often seems easier to forgo physical activities for other priorities. First and foremost, physical activity at any age should be fun because enjoyment is a strong motivator for continuing any behavior, as are social interactions that develop new friendships. For children, the joy of physical activity should be the centerpiece of sport and fitness programs. Aside from the necessity of keeping things fun, it is important to recognize that, in many respects, children are not simply small adults. The ways in which children and adults differ in their responses to physical activity and training must be considered in designing safe and effective training programs for children.

One example of the differences between adults and children is in designing training programs for children when there is often a large disparity between the ages of children and their maturity levels. Age and maturation are sometimes disconnected, especially when it comes to emotions and behavior. You know friends or children whom you consider to be more mature or less mature for their ages. But those judgments are made based on whether their emotional reactions or behaviors fit expectations for a particular age.

> By age two, most children will have already reached 50% of their adult height.

FIGURE 11.1 Growth, development, and maturation are defined differently but occur simultaneously during aging.

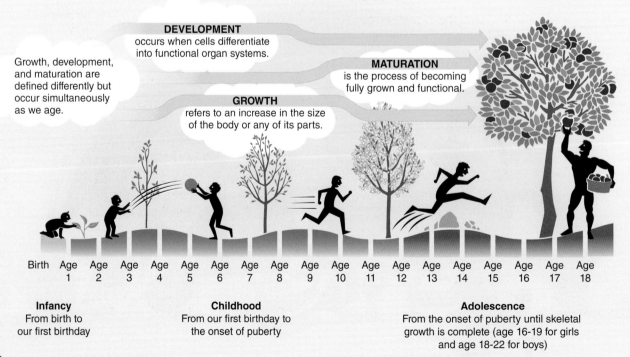

Growth, development, and maturation are defined differently but occur simultaneously as we age.

DEVELOPMENT
occurs when cells differentiate into functional organ systems.

MATURATION
is the process of becoming fully grown and functional.

GROWTH
refers to an increase in the size of the body or any of its parts.

Birth | Age 1 | Age 2 | Age 3 | Age 4 | Age 5 | Age 6 | Age 7 | Age 8 | Age 9 | Age 10 | Age 11 | Age 12 | Age 13 | Age 14 | Age 15 | Age 16 | Age 17 | Age 18

Infancy
From birth to our first birthday

Childhood
From our first birthday to the onset of puberty

Adolescence
From the onset of puberty until skeletal growth is complete (age 16-19 for girls and age 18-22 for boys)

From a physical perspective, maturity is determined with a little more objectivity. People mature physically (experience maturation) at slightly different rates from infancy (birth to the first birthday) through childhood and into adolescence, before finally reaching adulthood. (See figure 11.1.) At any given time in development, physical maturity is determined by chronological age, skeletal age, and stage of sexual maturation.

In some sports, age-group competition is a common way to attempt to have children and adolescents compete against other kids of similar maturity. In other sports, body weight is used to categorize competitors to make competition more fair. Rules of this sort can help level the playing field but cannot account for different levels of maturity. For example, 10- to 12-year-old swimmers vary dramatically in height, weight, sexual maturity, strength, endurance, and speed. And there can be similarly large differences in the maturity of 14-year-old and 18-year-old wrestlers in the same weight class. Although only so much can be done to have competitions fairly reflect the differences that occur during aging, it is important to keep those differences in mind when developing training programs.

Does Training Hurt or Help Children's Bones?

As with skeletal muscles and the heart, bone adapts to the stress imposed by regular exercise. Well-designed training programs, general play activities, and proper nutrition (adequate intake of calcium and vitamin D) stimulate adaptations that create stronger, healthier bones.

Most bones form from cartilage during fetal development, a process (*ossification*) that continues until the onset of adulthood. Bones grow as cartilage hardens into bone. The line of cartilage called the *epiphyseal plate* (but commonly known as the *growth plate*) indicates a bone that is still growing (figure 11.2). A bone that has stopped growing is considered *fused*. The growth plates in the bones of girls usually fuse a couple of years sooner than in boys due to female hormones that signal the growth plates to close.

Regular physical activity at any age benefits bone health, but that is especially true in children and adolescents. High-impact activities such as running and repeated jumping stimulate bone formation by exposing the bone to sufficient stress and strain to promote adaptations. *Bone mineral density*, an indicator of bone health and strength, peaks during a person's 20s and then slowly declines thereafter. Because of that slow decline in bone mineral density later in life, achieving a higher peak bone density is beneficial for younger people. Proper nutrition and exercise during childhood and adolescence create a greater peak bone density, an important factor in preserving healthy bones throughout life. In women, menopause causes an accelerated loss of bone, increasing the risk of *osteoporosis* in those who had low bone density earlier in life.

> Muscle mass typically peaks in girls between ages 16 and 20 and in boys between ages 18 and 25.

FIGURE 11.2 In children, the ends of long bones (such as the bones in the arms and legs) are made partly of cartilage. The bone grows as the cartilage hardens at the line called the growth plate or epiphyseal plate.

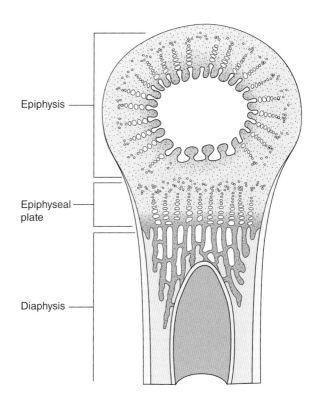

Epiphysis

Epiphyseal plate

Diaphysis

Development of the Nervous System in Children and Adolescents

Regular physical activity—whether in organized sports or just playing outside—requires a child's developing nervous system to adapt to various demands. These adaptations occur year after year as the brain and motor nerves undergo *myelination*. (See figure 11.3.) Myelination speeds nerve impulses and that means faster reaction times and more coordinated movements. Children who learn new movements and sports skills as their nervous systems are developing and myelination is taking place will be more proficient at those skills later in life and thereby less intimidated to participate in sports and fitness activities.

Blood pressure is related to body size and is lower in children than in adults.

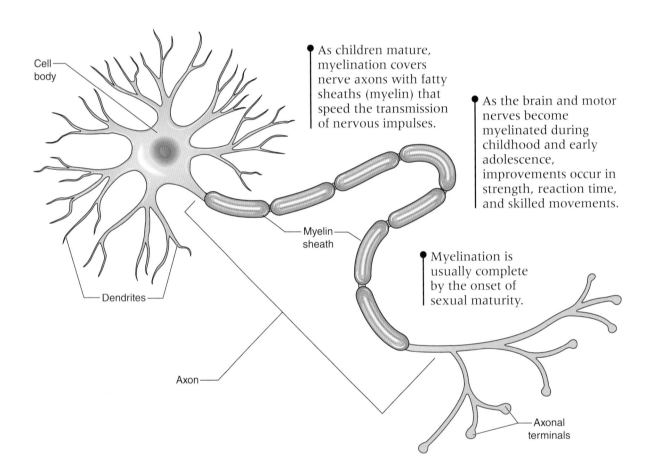

Cell body

As children mature, myelination covers nerve axons with fatty sheaths (myelin) that speed the transmission of nervous impulses.

As the brain and motor nerves become myelinated during childhood and early adolescence, improvements occur in strength, reaction time, and skilled movements.

Myelin sheath

Myelination is usually complete by the onset of sexual maturity.

Dendrites

Axon

Axonal terminals

FIGURE 11.3 The myelin sheath around nerve fibers develops during childhood and improves transmission of neural impulses.

Being good as a young athlete is no guarantee of being similarly good as an older athlete. A study of age-group swimmers showed that only a small percentage (<20%) of the fastest athletes at ages 17-18 were among the fastest when they were 10-12 years of age.

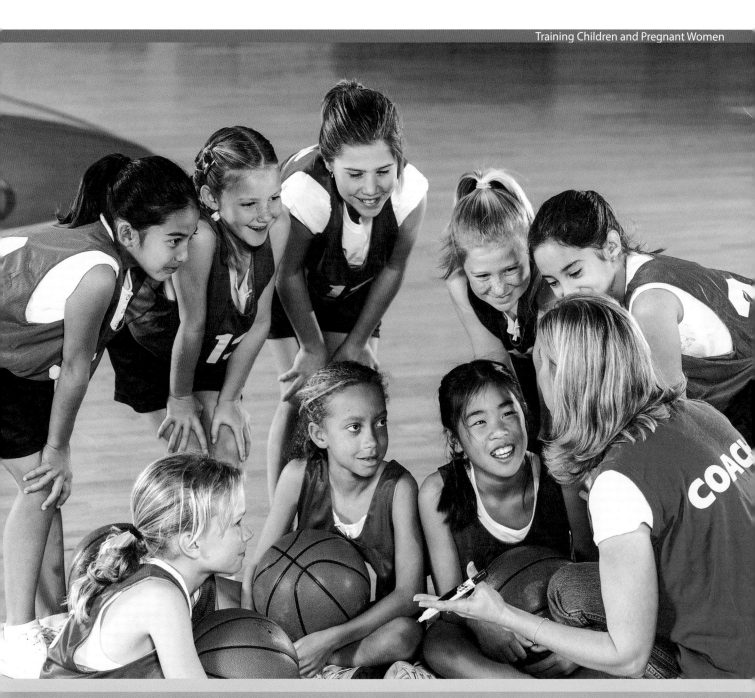

When Should Children Specialize in a Sport?

Regular physical activity helps children develop motor skills such as balance, agility, and coordination that are important in sports and helps establish a foundation of fitness-related skills important throughout life. For that reason, children should experience a variety of sports and physical activities so that they learn new skills and movement patterns and improve their fitness, responses that will benefit them throughout life. Research on 237 NBA players indicated that those who participated in multiple sports as kids played more NBA games, had longer careers, and were less likely to be injured compared to players who focused solely on basketball.

Motor skills—including sport-specific skills—improve rapidly through adolescence, another reason why it is important for children and teens to participate in a variety of activities. Skills gained early in life are skills that can be used throughout life.

Rugg, C. et al. 2018. The effects of playing multiple high school sports on National Basketball Association players' propensity for injury and athletic performance. *The American Journal of Sports Medicine.* 46(2):402-408.

Can Children Improve Strength With Training?

The short answer to this question is yes, children can increase their strength through proper training, including resistance exercise.

Strength increases during the maturation process because muscles naturally become larger and because myelination of the nervous system is completed around the time of sexual maturity. Bigger muscles result from the hypertrophy of muscle cells, not from *hyperplasia* (increased number of cells). Not surprisingly, puberty sparks a rapid increase in muscle strength in both boys and girls. As growth slows toward the end of adolescence, muscle strength plateaus unless physical labor or exercise routines stress muscles enough to stimulate the adaptations needed for increased strength.

Before puberty, increases in strength occur without any change in the size of muscles. Keep in mind that strength can increase by the recruitment of more motor units, as a result of improved coordination, and through the development of better sport-specific skills, none of which require an increase in muscle size. All the basic principles of strength training apply to children. However, extra care should be taken to develop proper strength training skills and prevent injury. See the blue sidebar for an overview of recommendations.

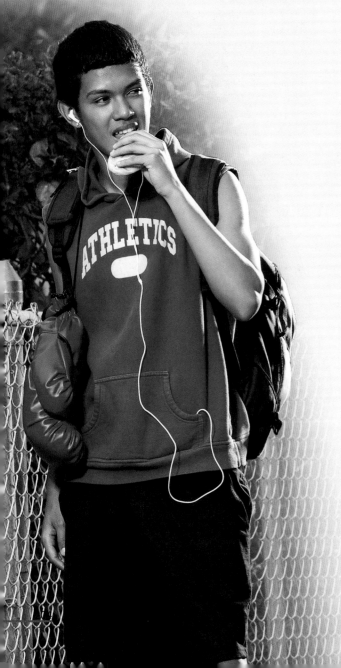

Performance Nutrition Spotlight

Children and teens who often skip breakfast before heading to school or to a morning practice are missing a great opportunity to aid their growth and development both academically and as athletes. It would be wonderful if all kids ate a nutritious, well-balanced breakfast, but the good intent of that wishful thinking is often lost on youngsters. Instead of trying to convince reluctant kids to eat a wholesome breakfast, first attempt to persuade them to eat or drink something—anything—to simply establish a habit of eating before they leave the house. Even a gulp of milk or a bite of an apple is better than nothing and those simple steps can eventually evolve into breakfast behaviors that come closer to ideal.

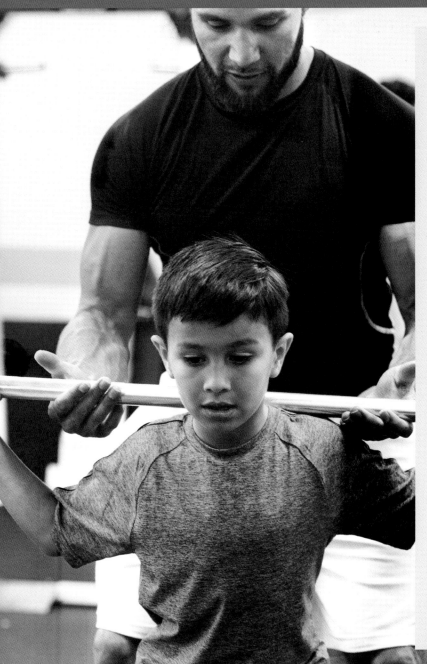

Recommendations for Strength Training in Children

- Proper exercise technique should always be the top priority, regardless of an athlete's age. This is particularly true with young athletes.
- The training area should be supervised by qualified adults and free of hazards.
- Progress from body-weight exercises to conventional strength training exercises using little to no weight to help kids learn proper technique. Technique development is especially important before puberty when there will be little change in muscle mass.
- Include exercises that strengthen muscles throughout the body.
- Keep training volume low (no more than 3 times per week), keep the exercises simple, and gradually increase the number of exercises in each session.
- Eventually teach all the basic exercise and lifting techniques, something that should be accomplished over years, not months.
- In teaching new techniques, always begin with little to no resistance.
- As kids reach puberty, which is begin to transition from general resistance exercises to sport-specific resistance exercises.
- After puberty, the volume and intensity of strength training can be gradually increased.

Should Children Diet?

As an increasing number of children become overweight or obese, there is no doubt that increasing daily physical activity is an important part of stimulating weight loss—and of preventing weight gain in the first place. Current guidelines call for children to engage in at least 60 minutes of physical activity each day. The American Academy of Pediatrics recommends that overweight children increase their daily physical activity (energy output) and modestly restrict their energy intake by choosing a balanced diet of healthy foods, in appropriate portions, to produce a gradual loss of body weight (e.g., 1 lb [0.5 kg] per week). It is best to recommend that parents consult a pediatrician or registered dietitian nutritionist (RDN) for guidance in helping their children lose fat weight.

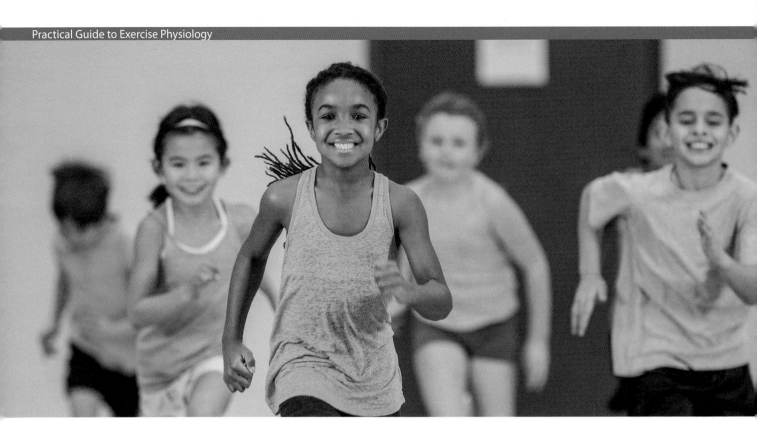

How Do Children Respond to Exercise?

Children can participate in virtually all types of exercise without undue risk to health as long as the limitations in their physiology are taken into consideration. For example, children have a limited capacity for anaerobic exercise because their muscles contain low levels of anaerobic (glycolytic) enzymes. For that and other reasons, high-intensity training should wait until adolescence (age 12 and older). Figure 11.4 illustrates how children respond to a single bout of exercise.

Should training programs be modified to account for how children adapt to training? The short answer is no. Although there are some differences between children and adults in the magnitude of the adaptations to training, children adapt to the stress of exercise training in similar ways compared to adults. In short, there is no reason to alter the principles of training program design covered in chapter 5. Here are the expected responses to training in children:

> $\dot{V}O_{2max}$ and running economy are lower in children than in adults.

- Children can decrease body weight and body fat with training, but their increase in lean body mass is less than in adolescents and adults.

- Muscle glycolytic capacity, PCr, and ATP levels all increase with training in children.

- Regular training has no effect on the height achieved in adulthood.

- Improvements in $\dot{V}O_{2max}$ in children range from 5% to 15%, compared to 10% to 20% in adolescents and adults.

- The improvement in $\dot{V}O_{2max}$ after puberty may be due to increases in stroke volume that occur as the heart grows.

$\dot{V}O_{2max}$ is lower in children than in adults, but increases progressively with age until the end of adolescence.

$\dot{V}O_{2max}$ will increase with training but those changes are relatively small compared to the changes that adults undergo. However, performance improvements in children can be large.

Children have lower **blood pressure** than adults because their bodies and hearts are smaller.

Even though blood pressure during exercise is lower in children, it does not limit blood flow to muscles because kids have less peripheral resistance.

Maximal **heart rate** is greater in children than in adults.

Because children have smaller hearts and smaller stroke volumes, their heart rates are higher than those of adults for similar levels of exercise.

Maximal **ventilatory volume** is lower in children than in adults.

Compared to adults' muscles, children's muscles are able to extract more oxygen from blood, another compensation for smaller stroke volumes.

Children have a larger ratio of **surface area** to mass than adults do, which means that children can gain or lose heat more quickly than adults.

Children have lower **movement economy** than adults do, but it improves steadily with training and age.

Children **sweat** less and acclimate more slowly to the heat than adults do.

Compared to adults, children have a lower **capacity for intense exercise** because of a lower glycolytic capacity. Consequently, children produce less lactic acid.

Children have less **muscle glycogen** and rely more on fat oxidation during exercise than adults do.

Children and adults have similar **levels of ATP and PC** in muscle cells, so brief bouts of intense exercise are not compromised in children.

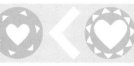

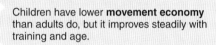

FIGURE 11.4   Although there are differences between children and adults in some of the physiological and metabolic responses to acute exercise, none of those differences prevents children from participating in virtually all types of exercise.

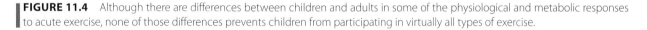

Are Dietary Supplements Safe for Children?

Should children and adolescents consume dietary supplements? It is impossible to provide a blanket recommendation for supplement consumption by children and adolescents because there are more than 50,000 dietary supplements on the market, most of which do not have adequate evidence of safety or efficacy, especially in children and adolescents. Children and adults alike should be able to consume all the essential nutrients by eating a balanced diet rich in fruits, vegetables (including *pulses*—beans, peas, lentils), lean meats and fish, whole grains, nuts, seeds, and dairy products. A low-dose multivitamin and mineral supplement can help ensure an adequate intake of micronutrients if parents are concerned that their children are not always eating as healthy a diet as they would like. Unless recommended by a physician, there is normally no reason that children and adolescents should consume other dietary supplements, and that is particularly true for sport supplements such as creatine and beta-alanine.

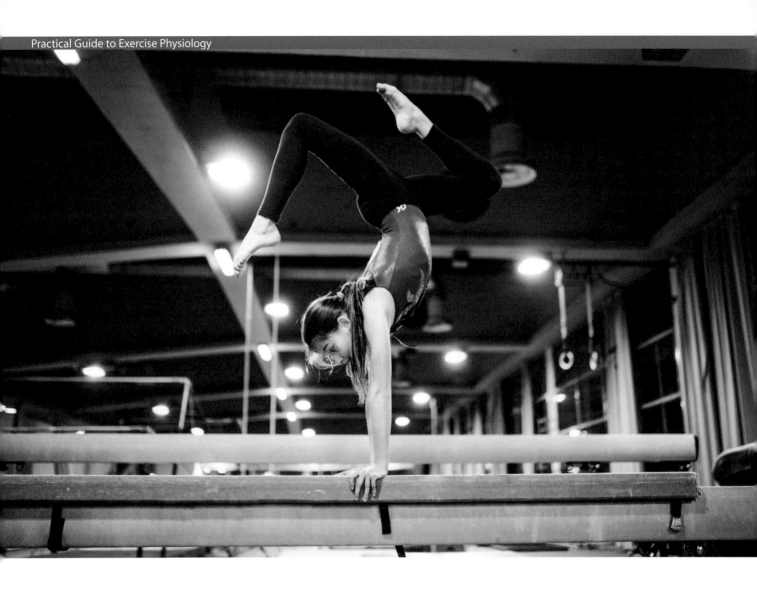

What Are the Safe Limits for Training in Children?

Not much is known about how endurance training affects children (12 years of age and younger) because the topic has not been well studied. It is obvious that children can adapt to endurance training and can achieve significant improvements in performance in sports such as swimming, running, and cycling. There are unresolved concerns about how training in children might affect overall growth, bone development, onset of menses, risk of orthopedic injuries, socialization, and psychological development. In those regards, research has lagged behind practical experience because in many sports, swimming being a good example, young children often train for hours on a daily basis without any documented issues with growth and development. However, in designing training programs for children, you need to take care to ensure that training and nutrition can best augment natural growth and development, both physically and psychologically.

A general rule is that children can begin to train like adults in late adolescence (age 15 and older), toward the end of their musculoskeletal growth stage when their bodies are better able to withstand the intensity, duration, and frequency of vigorous training. There is no doubt that some young gymnasts, swimmers, and runners undertake training programs that many adult athletes would find impossible to handle, seemingly without any long-term negative consequences. It is also true that many young athletes burn out from the physical and psychological demands of hard training. This is a good example of where the art and experience of coaching are often the best guides in making decisions about how hard, how long, and how often children should train, in part because there is not yet enough scientific information on which to base such decisions.

Performance Nutrition Spotlight

It is recommended that caffeine consumption in children be limited to 2.5 milligrams per kilogram of body weight per day, which is the equivalent of roughly 1 milligram of caffeine per pound of body weight per day.

Menstruation, Hormones, and Exercise Performance

Although still a matter of some debate among sport scientists, menstruation does not seem to affect physiological and metabolic responses to exercise, nor does it influence sport performance, unless the menstrual symptoms are so severe as to restrict exercise. In fact, world records across sports have been set during every phase of the menstrual cycle. There is no doubt that menstruation and its hormonal underpinnings influence body temperature, fluid balance, and metabolism, but the combined effects of those changes on performance are less clear.

The age at which menstruation begins (*menarche*) does not seem to be affected by the type of sport. Small, lean girls in any sport are most likely to have delayed menarche because of low body fat. Disturbances in the menstrual cycle (e.g., infrequent or no periods) in athletes and nonathletes alike can occur with caloric restriction. This energy deficit can be exaggerated in athletes because of the large daily energy outputs associated with training. Energy deficits in female athletes can affect long-term health of bones and reproductive organs because of reductions in estrogen, progesterone, luteinizing hormone, and thyroid production along with compromised intakes of calcium, vitamin D, and protein.

One of the reasons that girls are at increased risk of injury to the anterior cruciate ligament (ACL) compared to boys is that testosterone strengthens ligaments, whereas estrogen (and perhaps other hormones) weakens ligaments. When the fibroblasts in ligaments are exposed to testosterone, they increase their production of collagen proteins, strengthening the ligaments. Estrogen exposure decreases collagen production. Other factors that increase the risk of ACL injuries in girls include differences in quadriceps and hamstring strength as well as differences in the biomechanics of how girls land after jumping. For these reasons, training in young girls should stress leg-strength exercises and proper landing techniques, especially in sports such as basketball, soccer, softball, lacrosse, and hockey.

Should Women Exercise During Pregnancy?

The American College of Sports Medicine (ACSM) encourages women to remain physically active throughout pregnancy as long as there are no health-related contraindications. Regular exercise during normal pregnancies reduces health risks for both mother and baby, and the physiological changes that accompany pregnancy—such as increased blood volume—help support continued physical activity. Training programs for pregnant women should be modified to suit each woman's interests, abilities, and symptoms, as well as to reduce the chances of hypoxia, hyperthermia, and restricted carbohydrate supply to the developing baby and prevent possible miscarriage, low birth weight, or abnormal development

Following are general guidelines for exercise for pregnant women, but women should always consult their physicians for individual advice on the proper exercise program.

Pregnant women are advised to consume an extra 300 Calories (kcal) per day to support the developing fetus, so women who train during pregnancy should pay particular attention to adequate energy intake.

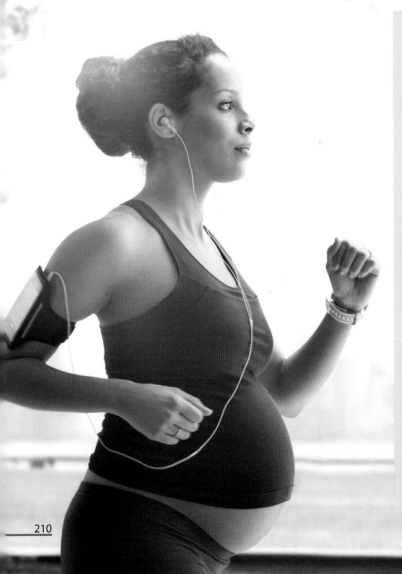

Training Guidelines for Pregnant Women

- Recommended exercise includes activities that use large muscle groups, such as walking, cycling, and swimming.
- During the first trimester, exercise can start at 15 minutes per day 3 days per week, or as comfort and symptoms dictate.
- After the first trimester, exercise should be limited to 30 minutes per day 4 days per week at a moderate intensity (e.g., heart rate less than 155 bpm).
- Avoid dry-land supine exercise after the 16th week of pregnancy to reduce the risk of venous obstruction.
- Avoid hot environments and remain well hydrated.
- Strength training can be continued during pregnancy using resistance that results in modest fatigue after 12 to 15 reps.
- Never restrict breathing during exercise (i.e., no Valsalva maneuvers).
- Contraindications for exercise during pregnancy include anemia, diabetes, bronchitis, obesity, anorexia, hypertension (*preeclampsia*), joint pain or injury, uncontrolled seizures, heart and lung disease, bleeding, and premature labor.
- Exercise can resume about a month after vaginal delivery and 2 months after cesarean section.

Chapter Summary

- During childhood and adolescence, growth and maturation do not always occur at similar rates.
- Physical activities that place stress and strain on bones (e.g., running and jumping) aid in bone formation and strength.
- Peak bone mineral density typically occurs before age 30 and declines slowly thereafter, with accelerated bone mineral loss accompanying menopause.
- Developing strong bones early in life helps prevent osteoporosis later in life.
- The myelination of nerves continues throughout childhood and is usually complete by the time of sexual maturity.
- Prior to puberty, the emphasis of strength training should be on developing proper technique using very light weights.
- Children have the metabolic capacity (adequate muscle cell PCr and ATP content) to sprint short distances but are limited in their ability to tolerate intense interval training because of lower glycolytic capacity.
- Training induces adaptations in children and adolescents that are directionally similar to those that occur in adults.
- Delayed menarche in female athletes is most likely due to small body size, low body fat, and energy restriction rather than to the rigors of a particular sport.
- Regular physical activity during pregnancy reduces health risks for both the mother and baby.
- Avoid physical activity during pregnancy that might limit oxygen or carbohydrate supply, restrict blood flow, or overheat the developing baby.

Review Questions

1. Differentiate the terms development, growth, and maturation.
2. Identify the change that is primarily responsible for bone growth.
3. Explain the relationship between myelination and the development of sports skills in children.
4. Describe two differences in how children and adults respond physiologically to exercise.
5. Discuss two exercise-related precautions pregnant women should consider.

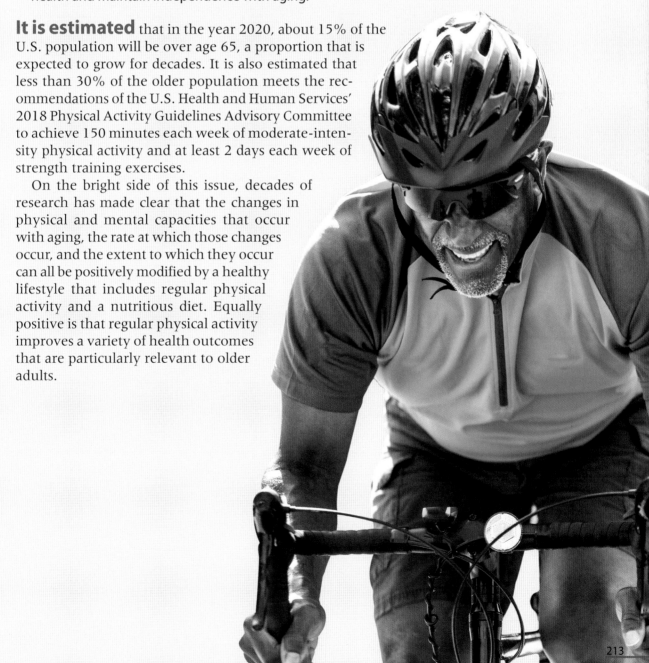

CHAPTER TWELVE

Training Older Adults

Objectives

- Understand how regular physical activity throughout life helps reduce the risk of all-cause mortality and extends the healthspan.
- Learn how aging affects the health and physical capacities of older adults.
- Appreciate the many benefits of strength training and their ability to improve health and maintain independence with aging.

It is estimated that in the year 2020, about 15% of the U.S. population will be over age 65, a proportion that is expected to grow for decades. It is also estimated that less than 30% of the older population meets the recommendations of the U.S. Health and Human Services' 2018 Physical Activity Guidelines Advisory Committee to achieve 150 minutes each week of moderate-intensity physical activity and at least 2 days each week of strength training exercises.

On the bright side of this issue, decades of research has made clear that the changes in physical and mental capacities that occur with aging, the rate at which those changes occur, and the extent to which they occur can all be positively modified by a healthy lifestyle that includes regular physical activity and a nutritious diet. Equally positive is that regular physical activity improves a variety of health outcomes that are particularly relevant to older adults.

What Changes With Aging?

A variety of changes occur during the aging process, as shown in figure 12.1. For some older adults, these changes become so significant that they interfere with the *activities of daily living* (ADL), simple tasks such as opening jars, lifting groceries, walking stairs, rising easily from a chair, and maintaining balance. Although some changes with age are unavoidable, most can be positively affected by a nutritious diet, regular physical activity, and proper training. In this context, *physical activity* refers to any body movement that expends energy—activities such as walking, climbing stairs, working in the yard, playing with grandchildren, or bicycling around the neighborhood. In contrast, *exercise* encompasses structured, planned, repeated activities with the goal of improving some aspect of physical fitness. Regardless of that distinction, the vast majority of older adults in the U.S. lead lives that are deficient in both physical activity and exercise.

For example, body weight tends to increase in many people after age 25 because of a reduction in daily physical activity and an increase in energy intake. After age 65, body weight tends to gradually decrease in many older adults as appetite and physical activity decline and muscle mass is lost at an accelerated rate. However, loss of muscle mass can begin decades earlier in those who lead sedentary lifestyles.

From a sport perspective, performance capacity is greatest during a person's 20s through her early to mid-30s and begins to decline slowly thereafter. The decline in distance and sprint performance averages about 1% each year after

Health Benefits of Regular Physical Activity for Older Adults*

- Improved ability to accomplish activities of daily living
- Improved sleep quality, functioning, and feelings of well-being
- Improved perceived quality of life
- Increased loss of fat weight
- Increased prevention or minimization of weight gain
- Reduced risk of falls and related injuries
- Increased prevention or remediation of frailty and sarcopenia
- Reduced risk of cardiovascular diseases
- Reduced risk of osteoarthritis
- Improved physical function in multiple sclerosis
- Improved memory, processing speed, attention, and executive function (task initiation, emotional control)
- Reduced symptoms of depression
- Reduced symptoms of anxiety
- Reduced risk of dementia
- Reduced risk of breast, colon, bladder, endometrial, esophageal, kidney, lung, and stomach cancers
- Reduced risk of (and part of treatment for) diabetes
- Reduced risk of (and part of treatment for) hypertension
- Improved physical function in Parkinson's disease
- Improved physical function in spinal cord injury

*Based on 2018 Physical Activity Guidelines Advisory Committee Scientific Report; https://health.gov/paguidelines/second-edition/report.aspx

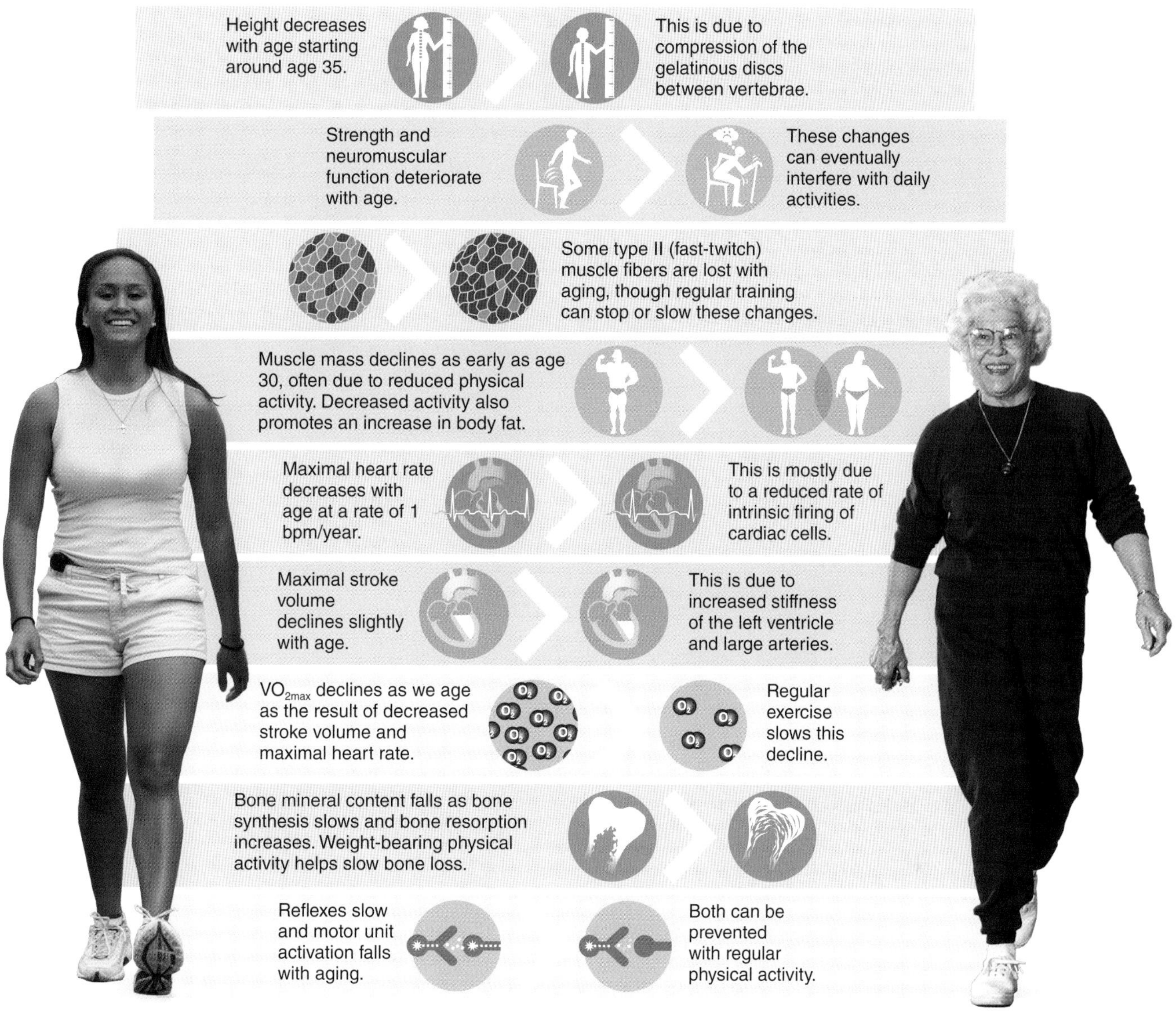

FIGURE 12.1 A variety of changes occur in the body during aging. In sedentary people, the negative changes to health and fitness are often more pronounced than they are in older adults who have remained physically active.

age 25. After age 70, the rate of decline increases to 2% per year for reasons that remain unclear. The reduction in performance capacity is associated with the aging-related declines in strength and aerobic capacity. Even though a decline in performance capacity is inevitable with aging, the rate of that decline can be slowed by regular training. In fact, sport performance in some older adults can equal or exceed that of many younger adults.

Performance Nutrition Spotlight

Older adults should strive to consume diets that are sufficient in energy (calories), protein, vitamins D and B_{12}, omega-3 fatty acids, and antioxidants provided by whole foods (fruits and vegetables). A nutritious diet and regular physical activity help preserve muscle mass and neuromuscular function with aging.

How Can Exercise Training Benefit Older Adults?

Older women and men respond to training similarly to younger people, increasing performance capacity along with physiological and metabolic function. For that reason, it is not unusual for 60-year-old athletes to have performance capacities that are greater than the capacities in people half their age. The ability to maintain impressive performance capacities occurs despite the fact that maximum cardiac output declines with age because both maximum heart rate and maximum stroke volume fall with age, as does blood flow to the arms and legs.

One of the challenges in establishing the effects of aging on physical fitness and performance is that it is difficult for scientists to separate the effects of aging from the effects of decades of relative inactivity in sedentary individuals. The same complication is true with older adults who have remained active but have reduced training intensity and duration over the years. Regardless, the good news is that proper training clearly improves all facets of physical capacity, including muscle mass, strength, endurance, aerobic capacity, agility, balance, coordination, flexibility, and anaerobic capacity.

> After age 60, the failure rate for opening the lid on a jar rises substantially. Loss of strength and muscle mass are due to decreased anabolic signaling, increased muscle catabolism, reduced physical activity, and inadequate protein intake.

The Strong Live Long

After age 40, sedentary individuals lose an average of 1% of their muscle mass each year (a range of 0.5-1.2% per year) along with a loss in strength that averages 3% per year. This loss of muscle mass is not unusual; all mammals experience something similar as they age. But when the loss of muscle mass and strength become so severe that muscular weakness interferes with the activities of daily living, there is a substantial negative impact on health care, living conditions, illnesses, and injuries. The severe loss of muscle mass and functional strength associated with aging and a sedentary lifestyle is called *sarcopenia*, a word coined in 1988 that means "poverty of flesh" in Greek. Sarcopenia occurs as a result of the loss of motoneurons and their associated motor units, combined with an increase in muscle protein breakdown and a decrease in muscle protein synthesis, leading to gradual decline in muscle mass and strength.

Protein synthesis in the muscle cells in older adults is less sensitive to dietary protein intake and to the normal stimulation of exercise. This *anabolic resistance* is one characteristic of aging muscle that predisposes many older adults to sar-

Performance Nutrition Spotlight

In addition to helping support muscle strength and mass in older adults, diets higher in protein (e.g., 1 g of protein per lb of body weight per day [0.5 g per kg BW per day]) are associated with greater weight loss, more fat loss, and better protection of lean body mass.

copenia. *Dynapenia* is the term that refers to inordinate muscular weakness. Fortunately, regular training and physical activity in general can substantially reduce the rate at which muscle mass, strength, and neuromuscular function are lost, even in very old adults (e.g., >90 years of age).

Figure 12.2 shows a striking example of the effect of strength training on muscle mass in later middle age. Strength training can also slow the loss of type II muscle fibers, and physical activity that incorporates weight-bearing exercises such as running and jumping (impact exercise) helps slow bone loss. Reducing the loss of muscular strength, muscle mass, and bone mass during aging is critical in maintaining the ability to live independently, decreasing the incidence of accidental falls, promoting more rapid recovery from injury and illness, and improving the overall quality of life.

With age, the normal close relationship between muscle mass and muscle strength is altered. Many older adults lose substantial muscle mass as they age, but if properly trained, can maintain sufficient muscle strength to preserve func-

FIGURE 12.2   Scans of the upper arms of three 57-year-old men of similar body weights. The white ring is bone, the gray area is muscle, and the black area is subcutaneous fat.

Reprinted, by permission, from W.L. Kenney, J.H. Wilmore, and D.L. Costill, *Physiology of Sport and Exercise*, 7th ed. (Champaign, IL: Human Kinetics, 2020), 66.

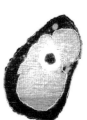

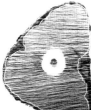
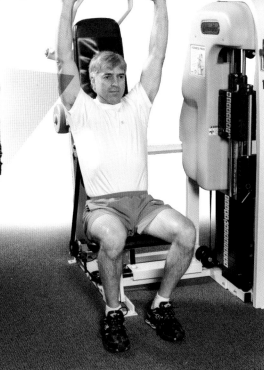

Untrained   Swim trained   Strength trained

Performance Nutrition Spotlight

After retirement, many older adults move to warmer climates where staying well hydrated can be challenging. Being even slightly dehydrated day after day can impair cognitive function and increase the risk of chronic kidney disease.

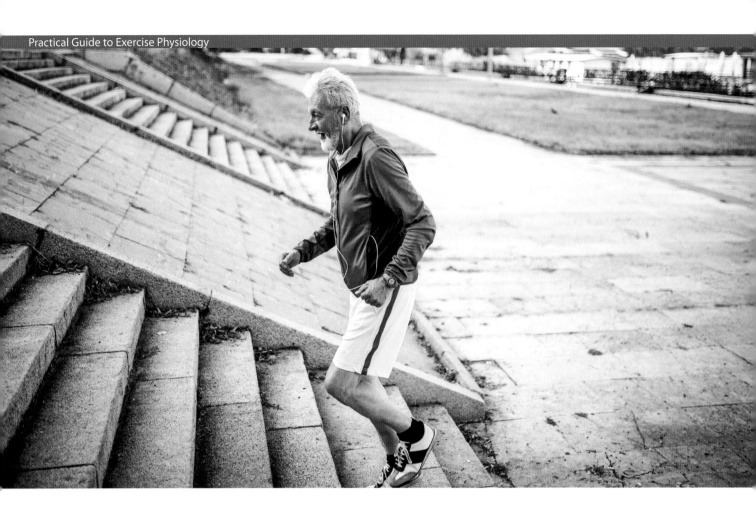

tional capacity and independence. It is also important that older adults maintain muscle endurance because leg muscles that fatigue quickly increase the risk of falling. Along the same lines, training that improves muscular power and the rate of force production not only reduces the risk of falls but helps older adults effortlessly rise from chairs, climb stairs, and improve their walking speed. Improved strength in older adults can result from positive changes in muscle mass and, perhaps more important, adaptations in the nervous system.

Proper strength training improves an older adult's ability to voluntarily recruit and activate the appropriate muscles, deactivate the appropriate antagonistic muscles, and better synchronize synergistic muscles. Improvements in muscle strength, endurance, and power in older adults prolong the ability to live independently, accomplish activities of daily living, recover more quickly from illness and injury, and reduce the risk of falls.

Falls in older adults can have catastrophic consequences whenever fall-related injuries result in even temporary immobility. The "*catabolic crisis*" that can follow fall-related injuries and immobility often sparks a rapid onset of sarcopenia and subsequent frailty, increasing the risk of an early death. Regular physical activity—including strength training—reduces fall risk in older adults by 30% to 40%, along with a 40% to 65% reduction in the risk of severe injuries from falling. In addition to at least two sessions of strength training each week, older adults should engage in *multicomponent physical activities* such as yoga, tai chi, team sports, dancing, handball, tennis, and pickleball—activities that develop stamina, strength, flexibility, balance, agility, and coordination. Such activities are better than strength training alone at improving overall functional performance in older adults.

Endurance training has little impact on the loss of muscle mass with age. Only strength training preserves muscle mass with age. However, endurance training does help slow the decline in $\dot{V}O_{2max}$ with age (figure 12.3). Older adults who begin aerobic exercise training usually experience the same 10% to 20% increase in $\dot{V}O_{2max}$ as younger individuals. Because maximal heart rate declines with increasing age and cannot be increased with training, improvements in $\dot{V}O_{2max}$ occur as a result of increases in stroke volume and a-$\dot{V}O_{2diff}$ (due to increases in oxidative enzyme activity in muscle cells).

Being physically fit also lowers the risk of heart attack (*myocardial infarction*) and improves the outcome when a heart attack does occur. Immediately following a heart attack, *ischemia-reperfusion injury* to cardiac muscle cells (and cells in other tissues that may have been temporarily deprived of oxygen) can occur as damaged, oxygen-starved cells are suddenly exposed to a higher blood oxygen content, resulting in inflammation and oxidative damage. Regular physical activity reduces the death of cardiac muscle cells following a heart attack and lowers the incidence of potentially dangerous heart *arrhythmias*. Aerobic training and HIIT are superior to strength training alone at increasing the number of blood vessels, improving the function of those vessels, and providing antioxidant protection for cardiac cells.

> Physical activity helps keep mitochondria young. In addition, some of the myokines released from active muscles appear to promote neurogenesis in the brain and improve memory.

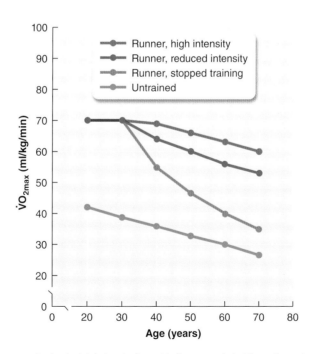

FIGURE 12.3 Runners who had a high level of aerobic fitness early in life and continue regular training as they age maintain a high level of fitness, even though they have a gradual overall decline in $\dot{V}O_{2max}$. Even if runners reduce intensity or stop training as they age, their fitness remains higher than that of people who had never trained.

Reprinted by permission from W.L. Kenney, J.H. Wilmore, and D.L. Costill, *Physiology of Sport and Exercise*, 6th ed. (Champaign, IL: Human Kinetics, 2015), 471.

Regular physical activity lowers the risks associated with heat and cold exposure. Heat stress in particular can be a problem for older adults, especially for those who are ill or at a very low level of fitness. When older adults are exposed to heat stress, blood flow to the skin and sweating are less than in younger adults, causing core temperature to rise more quickly. Fortunately, aerobic training can improve blood flow to the skin, increase sweating, and enhance the distribution of blood flow among skin, active muscles, and internal organs. These adaptations improve heat tolerance in older adults. With cold exposure, the blood vessels of the skin constrict less in older adults; because muscle mass is typically lower, older adults have a reduced ability to generate and retain metabolic heat.

These changes make older adults—especially the elderly—more susceptible to the cold. Adding more clothing when exercising outdoors and making other minor accommodations may be necessary to compensate for these age-related declines. Exposure to altitude poses the same challenges for older adults as for their younger counterparts and adaptations to altitude do not appear to be hampered with aging.

Low bone mineral density in swimmers and cyclists appears to be due to increased bone resorption (minerals move from bone into the blood) during training along with a lack of adequate stress and strain to stimulate bone formation. Weight-bearing activities are better for bone health because bones are exposed to more stress and strain, stimulating bone-building osteocyte activity.

Performance Nutrition Spotlight

The muscle cells of older adults become less sensitive to the amino acids supplied by the diet (anabolic resistance), so muscle protein synthesis tends to be lower compared to younger adults. For that reason, older adults should consume 40 grams of high-quality protein after exercise to optimize muscle protein synthesis.

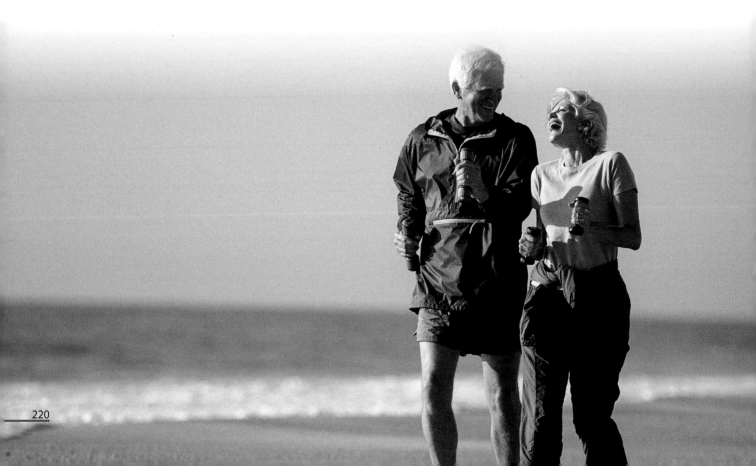

What Considerations Should Be Part of Training for Older Adults?

There are a variety of considerations that should be part of the general framework used to create and tailor training programs for older adults.

Considerations in Designing Training Programs for Older Adults

- Training programs for older adults should emphasize all aspects of physical fitness, including basic aerobic conditioning; exercises to improve muscular strength and mass; and activities that enhance flexibility, balance, and agility.

- Ideally, older adults should complete at least 150 minutes of moderate physical activity (e.g., brisk walking) each week, plus a minimum of two sessions of some sort of strength training designed to work all the major muscle groups.

- For those able to tackle more vigorous activity, attempt to complete at least 75 minutes of activity similar in intensity to jogging or running plus strength training twice each week.

- Older adults can also make use of HIIT as a way to improve aerobic fitness.

- Even short bouts of brisk stair climbing during the day (e.g., 20 sec of climbing followed by 2 min of rest, repeated three times) have been shown to improve aerobic capacity if done regularly (e.g., 3 days per week). Many older adults may find this kind of *"activity snack"* a convenient way to increase their physical activity and improve their overall fitness.

- Walking, bicycling, swimming, and other activities of a continuous nature are good starting points for improving aerobic capacity. With all activities, intensity is more important than duration at improving physical function and health outcomes. For example, research shows that walking speed should be greater than 2 mph (3 km/hr) to reap the associated health and fitness benefits.

- Simple body-weight exercises such as wall push-ups, toe stands, seated knee extensions, standing knee curls, supine pelvic tilts, and prone back extensions are examples of exercises that can improve functional capacity and muscular strength. These exercises can help older adults prepare for more strenuous resistance training with exercise bands, free weights, and other equipment or simply be a way to continue exercising at home.

- Fitness classes of any sort, including yoga and tai chi, are also appropriate for suitably motivated older adults.

- Older adults who are unaccustomed to strength training should begin with light weights to help develop proper exercise technique and begin to stimulate the muscle and connective tissue restructuring required for introducing progressive-overload training.

- Strength training for older adults should mimic movements used in their daily activities. For that reason, using weighted bags, elastic bands, and dumbbells rather than barbells is recommended.

- Older adults new to strength training or those who have not strength trained in decades may find continued success in terms of strength gains and compliance to the training regimen by exercising at an RPE of less than 8 on a 0-to-10 scale, where 10 is "extremely hard" and 8 is "hard."

- In addition to improving muscle strength and functional capacity, strength training can also help improve the aerobic capacity of older adults, particularly those adults who do little aerobic exercise.

- Multicomponent activities help improve agility, balance, and coordination, which are three characteristics that are not much improved by either endurance or strength training.

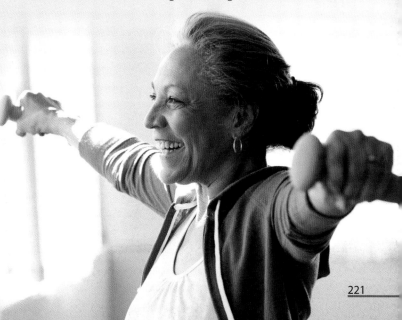

Chapter Summary

- In sedentary individuals after age 40, the decline in aerobic capacity and neuromuscular function (e.g., muscle mass, strength, motoneuron activation) approximates 1% to 2% each year.
- The gradual reduction in aerobic capacity is largely a result of lower maximal cardiac output brought about by lower maximal heart rate and stroke volume.
- Loss of neuromuscular function with aging is due to less motoneuron recruitment, increased muscle catabolism (decreased muscle protein synthesis, increased muscle protein breakdown), inadequate dietary protein intake, and reduced physical activity.
- With proper training, older adults can improve all aspects of physical fitness, although not to the levels achievable when they were younger.
- Sarcopenia among the elderly increases morbidity and mortality, but can be reversed with proper diet and exercise.
- For older adults who are not able to meet the current Physical Activity Guidelines for weekly exercise, brief bouts of activity such as stair climbing or brisk walking done on a regular basis (e.g., 3 days per week) can also confer benefits to fitness and health.
- Multicomponent physical activities that engage many muscle groups and require whole-body movements improve overall fitness and significantly reduce the risk of falling.

Review Questions

1. Summarize how strength, power, endurance, and muscle mass change as we age.
2. Identify the general type of physical activity that reduces the risk of falling in older adults.
3. Describe the relationship between exercise intensity and duration as it applies to improving fitness and health outcomes in older adults.
4. Explain two reasons for the loss of neuromuscular function with aging.
5. Define sarcopenia and describe how it can affect the health of older adults.

INDEX OF COMMON QUESTIONS FROM CLIENTS

General Physiology

What makes a muscle contract? (chapter 1)

How do nerves talk to muscles? (chapter 1)

Why do muscles feel tight when I stretch? (chapter 1)

Why are some people better at sprinting while others are better at endurance activities? (chapter 1)

What causes the fatigue I feel when I exercise? (chapter 4)

Why am I sore the day after a workout? (chapter 1)

Does lactic acid really cause fatigue? (chapter 4)

What's the difference between aerobic and anaerobic metabolism? (chapter 2)

How does oxygen get into the bloodstream? (chapter 3)

What happens to my blood pressure when I exercise? Does blood pressure change with training? (chapter 3)

What separates great athletes from the rest of us? (chapter 1)

Is a loss of physical ability with aging inevitable? (chapter 12)

What causes muscles to cramp? (chapter 1)

Program Design

Why does the same training program have different effects on different people? (chapters 1, 5, and 9)

What makes a good training program? (chapter 5)

If I stop training, will I lose all my gains in fitness? (chapter 5)

What is overtraining? (chapters 4 and 5)

How can I tell if I'm overtraining? (chapters 4 and 5)

Should I cross-train? (chapter 8)

When it comes to exercise, how are children different from adults? (chapter 11)

Should older adults exercise the same way that younger adults would? (chapter 12)

Should women exercise during pregnancy? (chapter 11)

Strength Training and Hypertrophy

What changes in my body with strength training? (chapter 1)

Why do muscles get stronger when I train? (chapter 1)

What makes muscles get bigger? (chapter 1)

What determines how much muscle I can gain? (chapter 6)

Will lifting weights give women big, bulky muscles? (chapter 6)

How often should I strength-train, and how many sets should I do? (chapter 6)

Can I build strength if I have only a short time for a workout? (chapter 6)

What kinds of equipment are best for strength training? (chapter 6)

Does muscle damage lead to increased strength? (chapter 1)

What are the effects of steroids on the body? (chapter 6)

Should endurance athletes strength-train? (chapter 9)

What supplements can I take to make me stronger? (chapters 1 and 6)

Endurance Training

What changes in my body when I do aerobic training? (chapters 1, 3, and 9)

Will aerobic fitness help my long-term health? (chapter 9)

Why do target heart rate and maximum heart rate get lower with age? (chapter 3)

What is $\dot{V}O_{2max}$? (chapter 3)

What is the relationship between $\dot{V}O_{2max}$ and endurance performance? (chapter 9)

What is the lactate threshold? (chapter 9)

How should I plan my training for an endurance event? (chapter 9)

How long will my endurance keep improving with training? (chapter 3)

Does endurance training give you more red blood cells? (chapter 9)

Is endurance important for athletes in team sports and nonendurance events? (chapter 9)

Why do East African runners win so many endurance events? (chapter 9)

How can I increase my muscle glycogen levels to improve endurance? (chapters 2 and 9)

Should endurance athletes do strength training? (chapters 6 and 9)

Anaerobic and Interval Training

What changes in my body when I do anaerobic training? (chapter 1)

What is interval training? (chapter 8)

How can I incorporate interval training into my workout? (chapter 8)

Should I do high-intensity interval training (HIIT)? How often? (chapter 5)

Can high-intensity interval training increase my endurance? (chapter 9)

What are the benefits of plyometric training? (chapter 8)

What is ballistic training? (chapter 8)

What does power really mean in athletic events? (chapter 8)

Can eating more protein help me improve my speed and power? (chapters 2, 6, and 8)

Is there a supplement I can take to reduce the negative effects of lactic acid? (chapter 8)

Weight Loss and Metabolism

Why do I have a difficult time losing weight? (chapter 7)

How many calories do I need to eat each day? (chapter 7)

What factors affect how many calories I burn in a day? (chapter 7)

How many calories do common physical activities burn? (chapter 7)

Does consuming calories during my workout defeat the purpose of trying to lose weight? (chapter 7)

Are low-calorie diets the best way to lose weight quickly? (chapter 7)

How can I lose fat without losing muscle? (chapter 7)

What's the best way to lose abdominal fat? (chapter 7)

What is the best exercise intensity for burning fat? (chapter 7)

Are there supplements I can take to increase fat burning? (chapter 7)

Will I burn more fat if I work out while fasting or on a low-carbohydrate diet? (chapter 7)

What does it mean to have a fast metabolism? How can I speed up my metabolism? (chapter 3)

What can I do to keep from losing muscle when I'm trying to lose fat? (chapters 6 and 7)

What is my resting metabolic rate? (chapter 7)

What is the oxygen deficit? Am I still burning extra calories after my workout? (chapter 3)

What are brown and beige fat? (chapter 7)

Should children diet? (chapter 11)

Safety and Environmental Issues

How can I avoid muscle cramps? (chapter 1)

Why is it so much harder to exercise when it is hot? (chapter 10)

What are the risks of exercising in the heat? (chapter 10)

What precautions should I take when exercising in the heat? (chapter 10)

Will acclimating to the heat improve my performance? (chapter 10)

Will pouring cold water on my head and neck help me stay cool during exercise? (chapter 10)

Why is hydration important? (chapters 2, 4, and 10)

Is it possible to drink too much? (chapter 2)

Should I drink during cold-weather activity? (chapter 10)

Why do I feel weaker when I'm at altitude? (chapter 10)

Is there less oxygen at higher altitudes? (chapter 10)

At what altitude is exercise performance affected? (chapter 10)

Does training at altitude improve performance at sea level? (chapter 10)

What changes should I make in my diet if I'm at altitude for more than a few days? (chapter10)

What exercises are safe for pregnant women? (chapter 11)

Does menstruation affect exercise performance? (chapter 11)

Is exercise training dangerous for children's growth? (chapter 11)

Should young athletes skip breakfast? (chapter 11)

Is it safe for children to strength-train? (chapter 11)

Can kids safely consume caffeine? (chapter 11)

Should adults reduce their exercise intensity with age? (chapter 12)

What changes with aging? (chapter 12)

What nutrients are most important for older adults? (chapter 12)

Why are older adults at risk of losing muscle mass? (chapter 12)

How can older adults reduce the risk of falling? (chapter 12)

Nutrition, Hydration, and Supplements

What do carbohydrate, fat, and protein do in my body? (chapter 2)

What happens to carbohydrate after I eat it? (chapter 2)

What happens to fat after I eat it? (chapter 2)

What happens to protein after I eat it? (chapter 2)

How much protein do I need to eat each day? (chapters 2 and 6)

Should I ingest protein after a workout? (chapters 2 and 6)

If I consume carbohydrate during my workout, will I avoid fatigue? (chapter 4)

Will energy drinks improve my performance? (chapter 2)

How much water do I need to drink each day? (chapter 2)

What are the effects of dehydration? (chapter 4)

Should I take high doses of vitamins and minerals? (chapter 2)

What does iron do in the body, and what are the effects of not getting enough iron? (chapter 3)

What dietary supplements can improve my speed and power? (chapter 8)

What supplements can help me lose weight? (chapter 7)

If muscles use ATP for energy, should I take an ATP supplement? (chapter 2)

INDEX

Note: The italicized *f* and *t* following page numbers refer to figures and tables, respectively.

A

abdominal fat 141
acclimation
    altitude 197
    cold 191
    heat 186, 186*f*
acetylcholine (ACh) 7*f*, 8
ACL injury risk 209
actin 5, 7*f*, 8, 11, 14
activities of daily living (ADL) 214
acute mountain sickness 197, 197*f*
adaptation
    aerobic training 14, 16-18, 22, 62, 95,
        164-165, 175*t*
    anaerobic training 18
    cardiorespiratory 56, 56*f*, 56*t*, 175*t*
    cardiovascular 62, 63*f*
    in children 206, 207*f*
    in competitive success 13*f*
    defined 106
    dehydration and 57
    factors affecting 14-15, 21
    fatigue role in 85
    functional protein production 100
    individuality in 93, 93*f*
    in muscle cells 14, 14*f*, 175*t*
    muscle damage and 20-21, 20*f*
    periodization and 98-99, 99*f*, 102-103,
        102*f*
    plyometric training 95
    for speed and power 150
    strength training 14, 19, 22, 95, 110-
        111, 110*f*, 113
adenosine triphosphate (ATP)
    depletion of 70*t*, 72, 72*f*
    energy pathways 32-34, 32*f*, 42, 42*f*, 43*t*
    metabolic flexibility and 150
    nutrient sources 30-31
    production and use 28-29, 28-29, 28*f*,
        28*f*, 34-35, 128
ADH (anti-diuretic hormone) 48-49
adipocytes 34
ADL (activities of daily living) 214
aerobic capacity. *See* $\dot{V}O_{2max}$
aerobic production of ATP 33, 56*f*
aerobic (endurance) training. *See also* endur-
    ance performance; $\dot{V}O_{2max}$
    adaptation to 14, 16-18, 22, 62, 95,
        164-165, 175*t*
    benefits of 164, 165*f*
    for children 208
    energy sources for 34
    general guidelines 173-175
    HIIT 94, 153, 154, 158, 176, 219
    nutrition for 166, 167
    in older adults 219, 219*f*
    power improvement in 148, 149*f*

strength training and 158, 177
$\dot{V}O_{2max}$ improvement and 168
agility 106
aging process. *See* older adults
alcohol (ethanol) 40*t*
aldosterone 49
alpha motor neurons 5, 6
altitude
    acclimation to 197
    atmospheric pressure and 53, 193, 193*f*
    effects on performance 194
    health risks of 197, 197*f*
    older adults and 220
    physiological adjustments to 194*f*, 195,
        195*f*
    training at altitude 67, 196
    of world cities 195*t*
altitude sickness 197, 197*f*
amino acids 38, 38*t*, 39*f*
anabolic hormones 119, 119*f*, 125
anabolic resistance 124, 216
anabolic steroids 24, 119, 119*f*
anaerobic capacity 176
anaerobic glycolysis 32*f*, 33, 43*t*
anaerobic threshold 59, 170, 170*f*
anaerobic training 18, 155. *See also* HIIT;
    speed and power
android obesity 141
anemia 55
anti-diuretic hormone (ADH) 48-49
antioxidants 167
arginine vasopressin 48-49
arrhythmias 219
athletic success
    in children 202
    determining factors 13*f*
atmospheric pressure 53, 193, 193*f*
ATP. *See* adenosine triphosphate (ATP)

B

ballistic training 157
banned substances
    EPO 66, 172
    steroids 24, 119, 119*f*
    in supplements 134, 160
basal metabolic rate (BMR) 57
beet juice 117
beta-alanine 156, 160, 207
Bikram (hot) yoga 190
biological variability 65
block periodization 98, 103, 106
blood and blood vessels
    adaptation in 56, 56*t*, 62, 63*f*
    dehydration and 57
    hematocrit 65, 172
    in oxygen transport 54-56, 54*f*, 55*f*, 56*f*
    vasoconstriction 191, 191*f*

blood doping 66, 172
blood flow restriction 67, 123
blood pressure 64, 202, 207*f*
BMR (basal metabolic rate) 57
body fat. *See* fat (body fat)
body image 141
body-weight exercises 221
bone health
    adaptation in 17, 18, 19
    in children 201, 201*f*
    in cyclists and swimmers 220
bone mineral density 201
brain function
    disruptions and fatigue 70*t*, 82, 82*f*
    glucose for 34
breakfast eating 140, 204
brown and beige fat 130-131

C

caffeine 42, 209
calcium
    in muscle contraction 7*f*, 8, 8*f*, 9, 81, 81*f*
    supplemental 45
calories
    daily needs 134-135, 135*t*
    in macronutrients 40*t*
    for pregnant women 210
    restriction of 134, 139, 140, 144, 209
    term use 41
carbohydrate
    breakdown and use of 30-31, 31*f*, 34-
        36, 35*f*, 36*f*, 40*f*, 43*t*
    caloric value 40*t*
    glycogen stores and 74-75
    for hypoglycemia prevention 85
    intake guidelines 128, 132, 166
    low-carbohydrate diets 144, 144*f*, 167
    in periodized nutrition 46
    for recovery 116
    respiratory exchange ratio 60-61
cardiac output
    adaptation in 56, 56*t*, 62, 63*f*
    aerobic capacity and 164-165
cardiorespiratory adaptation 56, 56*f*, 56*t*, 175*t*
cardiovascular adaptation 62, 63*f*
catabolic crisis 218
central fatigue 70-71, 71*t*, 73, 184
cherry juice 117, 156
children
    adaptation in 206, 207*f*
    athletic success in 202
    growth and maturation 200-202, 200*f*, 202*f*
    nutrition 204, 205, 207, 209
    obesity in 205
    sport specialization in 203
    strength training in 204-205
    training limits 208-209

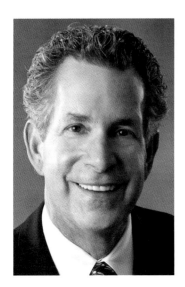

Bob Murray, PhD, FACSM, was a cofounder of the Gatorade Sports Science Institute (GSSI) and served as its director from 1985 to 2008. Murray oversaw a broad program of GSSI- and university-based research in exercise science and sport nutrition that set industry standards and consumer expectations for science-based product efficacy.

A native of Pittsburgh, Murray earned his BS and MEd degrees in physical education at Slippery Rock University. He was an assistant professor of physical education and head swimming coach at Oswego State University from 1974 to 1977 before earning his PhD in exercise physiology from Ohio State University. He was an assistant and associate professor of physical education at Boise State University from 1980 to 1985 before relocating to Chicago to begin work with Gatorade. In 2008, Murray founded Sports Science Insights LLC, a consulting group that helps clients with projects in exercise science and sports nutrition. An author of numerous publications in scientific texts and journals, and an invited speaker at professional meetings worldwide, Murray is a fellow of the American College of Sports Medicine and an honorary member of the Academy of Nutrition and Dietetics. Bob and his wife Linda live in Crystal Lake, Illinois.

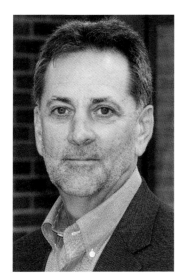

W. Larry Kenney, PhD, FACSM, FAPS, is the Marie Underhill Noll Chair in Human Performance and a professor of physiology and kinesiology at Pennsylvania State University. Dr. Kenney was awarded the prestigious Faculty Scholar Medal by Penn State for his research contributions. He has published more than 220 journal articles and dozens of book chapters on the topic of human responses to exercise, heat and cold stress, and dehydration as well as the biophysics of heat exchange between humans and the environment. He was continuously funded by National Institutes of Health (NIH) from 1986 through 2015, one of the longest-running R01 grants. Over the years, he has mentored 38 MS or PhD students along with 8 postdoctoral fellows and numerous undergraduate scholars.

Dr. Kenney is the primary author of *Physiology of Sport and Exercise*, a best-selling textbook in exercise physiology, now in its seventh edition; it has now been translated into 12 languages. He served as president of the American College of Sports Medicine from 2003 to 2004 and received the Citation Award from that organization in 2008. He is also a fellow of the American Physiological Society and was presented with the Adolph Distinguished Lectureship Award by that organization in 2017. He is the former chair of the Gatorade Sports Science Institute and serves on many scientific advisory panels, including Nike's Science Advisory Board.

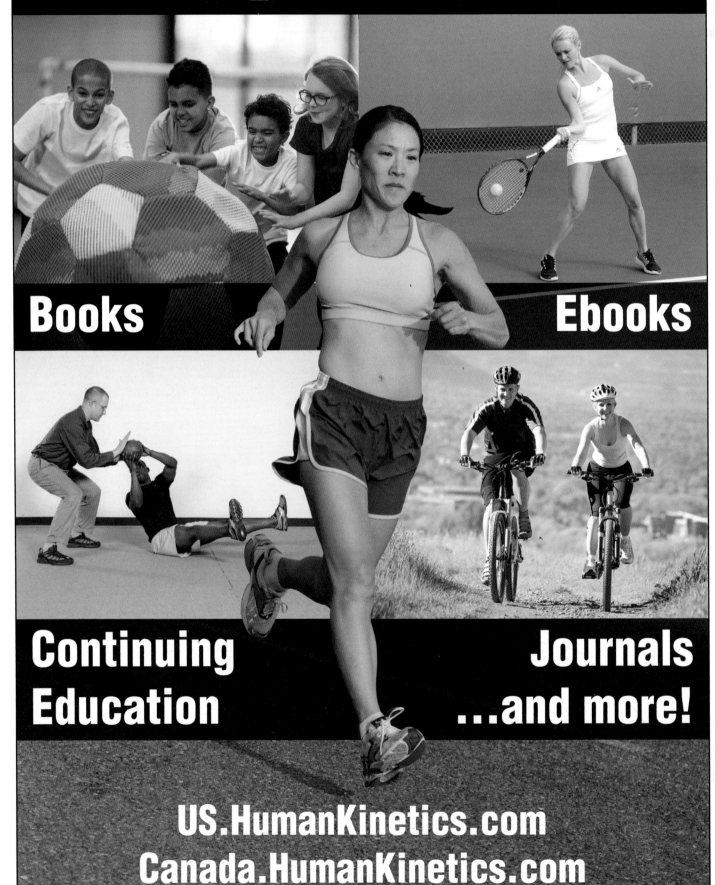